Living a Normal & Healthy Life After Renal (Kidney) Failure

PART TWO:
MY KIDNEY TRANSPLANTATION

Dr. Adeleke Eniola Oyenusi

CREDO

Weeping may endure for a night but joy cometh in the morning. —Psalms 30, Verse 5.

Living a Normal & Healthy Life after Renal (Kidney) Failure
My Kidney Transplantation, Part Two

Order this book online at www.trafford.com
www.kidneywelfare.com
or email orders@trafford.com

Most Trafford titles are also available at major online book retailers.

Printed in the United States of America.

ISBN: 978-1-4269-2674-7 (sc)
ISBN: 978-1-4269-7785-5 (e)

Trafford rev. 12/12/2013

Trafford PUBLISHING® www.trafford.com
North America & international
toll-free: 1 888 232 4444 (USA & Canada)
fax: 812 355 4082

Contents

PREFACE

My kidney Transplantation, Part 2, is a continuation of my first book, *Living a Normal and Healthy life after Renal (Kidney) Failure.* Here I will discuss at length my firsthand experience of this process.

With transplantation, a lot of things have to be taken into consideration; what to do and what to abstain from. Discovering how to prolong the life span of the kidney after transplantation made me think about writing part 2.

This book provides a comprehensive understanding of the kidney transplantation process, associated problems, and the positives for renal patients after successful transplantation, so that they can understand how the changes they will face will affect their lives, and to know that they are not alone with this challenge.

My aim is to enlighten the general public, and to create more awareness about kidney transplantation — one of the stages of living a normal and healthy life after renal (kidney) failure.

The following pages provide valuable information and education, for renal patients with little or no knowledge of kidney transplant procedures; much can be learned and gained from the book.

I encourage anybody with a renal condition, to get a copy of *Living a Normal and Healthy Life after Renal (Kidney) Failure.* It is encouraging and inspiring, and will restore confidence. Despite all limitations, hardship and setbacks, a person can still manage to live a normal and happy life after renal (kidney) failure.

Some religiously inclined people are of the opinion that we should not tamper with nature. They do not believe in organ transplants, likewise receiving donated blood when they are in need. Once an organ is damaged, they are of the opinion that we should not claim to be God by changing the organs, or accepting blood from other individuals. With kidney transplants there are many things one has to be prepared for, or adjust to.

Before my health problems, we were such a happy family. I was a very active person: taking my family to dine out, to cinemas, and the swimming pool, plus a lot of other indoor and outdoor activities. Since I fell sick, the anger, frustration and depression that kicked in made me forget about all these activities. I kept on thinking about death and loss of everything, including what is dear to me most — my family. Ten years of my life just went, in the blink of an eye. I want to make up for the lost years, especially for my kids, who experienced a lot of frustration, and saw me being carried away so many times, by an emergency ambulance.

I had my kidney transplant during my sixth year on dialysis, and can confirm that it was not easy during this time. At times I woke up in the middle of the night and cried until the following morning, not knowing what had happened to me. However, my determination, will power and the power of the Almighty helped me to bounce back, despite all limitations, against all odds. Self-discipline and consistency, backed up with prayers, paid off in the end.

I was eventually called on that fateful day for a kidney transplant. I was always optimistic, and never gave up, even at the most difficult times. I must admit I made some mistakes initially whilst adjusting to the reality of kidney failure but I soon learnt, and adjusted to conditions. I was ready to readjust my ways of life.

I kept on going, praying and believing that there would be a day that all my health suffering would come to an end. That day, the joyful life I used to have would be returned to me.

My desire is to help others who are in the same boat as I was. It is my hopes that any renal patients, their families, relatives or carers, reading this book, will be helped to more easily adjust to the new reality they face.

Transplantation is the total life-changing event that all renal patients dream about. It is a gift of a lifetime. However, having a kidney transplant is just the beginning of another journey. I wish to correct the misconception and misrepresentation of facts that when you are given a kidney transplant, "that is it," and all your health woes are over…

I am of the opinion that the more you know about kidney transplantation, the more you will be prepared to adjust, in order to take full advantage of the second chance of life which you have been given.

As a kidney transplant patient, as long as you stick to your medication and not forget to take your medication, especially the immunosuppressants, your kidney should be able to stand the test of time.

You cannot give up. You have to be optimistic, make the effort, be determined, stay focussed, be strong in mind, coupled with will power, and lastly back yourself up with prayers. Eventually, one day will be the day things will turn around for you. You will be given a new lease on life — another chance of living life, through your kidney transplant.

Keep the struggle alive and don't give up so easily. Do not lose hope; as they say: he who loses hope, loses everything. There are times when you get upset, fed up, depressed, and you feel ending it all. Remember that if you do give up, by committing suicide, you have lost the battle. Be patient. And I tell you from my experience, your patience will eventually pay off one day. Do not be in too much of a hurry to get the end result, just stay calm and be patient.

Please wait for your opportunity and moment, which I believe will definitely come, if you take stick with your treatment. Follow medical advice, be dedicated and have self-discipline.

I am of the opinion that it is a good idea to visit a doctor or a general practitioner regularly, at least once in a year, so as to avoid unforeseen health problems. A complete blood test can tell if the kidneys are functioning properly, or at their best.

NOTE: The experiences of kidney transplantation will be different for each individual.

ACKNOWLEDGEMENTS

First of all, I give honour and glory to God, for allowing me sail through the denial, anger, frustration, attempt to bargain, and depression that was part of the sickness. He saved and preserved my life to this day, allowing me to go through the health problems, hardship of high blood pressure, stroke and kidney failure for ten years. I was able to realise during the ten years of my sickness that if God says it is not yet time to die, nobody can take that life from you.

Secondly, because I had a cadaveric (organ donated by a dead person) kidney transplant, I would like to thank the families and relatives of the person that donated to me. I do acknowledge the pain of the relatives of my donor. They took that painful decision to help other people in need — like me — at a time when they were going through the painful emotions of their loved one's death. I honour and cherish what you have done for me, by giving me a second chance at life. I also pray that the soul of your loved one rests in perfect peace; Amen.

I wish to thank my own family, especially my wife, Gisele for her prayers, efforts, and understanding, and sharing the emotions of my sickness, coupled with the hardship, problems and depression that accompanied the sickness.

I thank my children, Kimberlyne, Kelvin and Kenneth, who for ten years, at a very tender age, knew only that their dad was being taken by the emergency ambulance to the hospital, when I had health crises. I hope that these ten years will not be in vain for you, but will make you much stronger, in order to be able to face the difficulties and challenges of life. May God Almighty bless you for me; Amen.

I also wish to specially thank the British government, which invented the NHS and social care, without which a lot of innocent lives could have been lost. I cannot express in words how humble and grateful I am for all your support and help. Whoever is in power at any time, may God continue to guide you and allow you to continue to know how to make things work.

My younger brother, Albert Adeniyi Oyenusi, (and wife Angela and Kingsley their son) provided immense support and help. You are a brother to be proud of. May the Lord in his mercy reward you with abundance of blessings; Amen.

Pastor Femi Oyejobi. Also my younger brother, his wife Hasannah and children, Mariam, Derby and Hannah who were also of immense help and support, both spiritually and morally.

I would like to thank my mother, Florence Omowunmi Oyenusi and my stepmother Adebola Oyenusi, for their constant prayers, concern and support.

I thank my aunties, Iyabo Sokunbi, Yetunde Sosanya, and uncles, Mr. Akinola Oyenusi, Deji Oyenusi and Soji Oyenusi for their support and prayers. My sisters, Adenike Oroge, Moji Adekunle, Iyabo Omobolanle Arojo, Sumbo Ohiosuman, Olaide Ladipo, Biodun and Toyin Adedeji, and brothers, Segun Oyenusi, Tunde Olanrewaju (Oyenusi), Adeyemi Oyenusi and Kola Adedeji were all of immense support.

I want to specially thank Dr. and Mrs. Ogunlowo for their contributions to my recovery. I also appreciate the role of Sonia Edgar, in helping make the book a reality.

I am also using this opportunity to thank Papa and Mama Nkunku, and all the family of my wife and friends— Magloire, Angel, Fanny, Yves, Makani, Nounou and Nino — for their concerns during my health problems. I appreciate the personal telephone call from Makani, and letters from Yves. I would like to thank Ani also for her concern and support.

I thank my friend Deacon Gbolahan Adekoya and Gbemi Adekoya his wife, for their support and prayers. Also Mr. Jimmy and Mrs. Anna Toriola, Mr. Adeniyi Odewole, Mr. Adeleke Akinsanya, Mr. Rafiu Ibrahim, Dr. Tunji Jolaosho, Mr. Ebenezer and Mrs. Omolola Hundeyin, Mr. and Mrs. Ananaba, Mrs. Suzan Ojiko-Adeyemi.

Members of the SAYUZNIKI: Paul Eboh, Olu Alaka, Innocent Chukwuemeka, Dr. Raheem Abaja, Dr. Razak Oyebade, Dr. Waheed Balogun, Dr. Raf Eke, Dr. Kelly Odigwe, Ama Oka Ama, Evangelist, Chioma Ojiofor, Dr. Osita, Dr. Tony Okoli, Emmanuel Ekanem, Mr. Davidson Osuagwu, Dr. Hogan Udo, Dr. Theo Madu, Kenneth Ideh, Dr. Nwosu Chinedu, Mr.Odulaja), Mr. Tunde Alao, Dr. (Rev) Oyebade, Dr. Yomi Sanni, Dr. Adefioye, Adegoke Fagbewesa, Rasak Abiwon, Dele Constant (Tajudeen Oladele), Dr. Daniel Oyetayo, Yemi Akinleye, Mr. Austin and Mrs Nwoma Achunene, Godwin Achunene, Mr.Chidi Agwamba, Mr. Hakeem Diko, Mr. Gbenga Aina, Mr. Johnson Akinwande.

Also I am grateful to my cousin Bola Oyinloye and her husband Pastor Oyinloye, Mrs. Funmilayo Oyefuga, Mrs Fela Adefule, Adetola Adeniyi Oyenusi, Adeolu Oyenusi, Adesoji Oyenusi, Adewunmi Oyenusi, Kunle Oyenusi, Dr. Adedoyin Oyenusi, Folarin Oyenusi, Niran Oyenusi, Mrs. Busola Olowa, Bolaji Oyejobi, Mrs. Yewande Ikutiminu, Tosin Oyenusi, Tolu Oyenusi, Wale Coker, and Lawon Opesanwo for their words of encouragement.

I want to thank Papa Charlie Mongo, and family: Mama Annie, Laeticia, Linda, Mimi, Keren, Price, Charlene Dino, Diki Mawete. Mama Beya, and family: Papa Don Pero, Trina, Diana, Dorcas, Mercy and Romeo.

My sincere thanks go to the members of the NHS Trust at the Royal London hospital, the doctors, nurses and domestics at the Paulin Ward, Devonshire Ward, Hanbury Dialysis Unit, the Low Dependence Unit (LDU), and the Dialysis Ward at the St Bartholomew's (Bart's) Hospital, Barbican. I appreciate the help of the renal dieticians of the Royal London Hospital, and Bart's. I do appreciate all your care.

I want to thank Professor Yakub, Dr. Islam Junaid, Dr. Gavin, Dr. Roberto Cacciola, and Dr. Carmelo Puliatti, Dr. Kulsoom Junejo, and Dr. Thurasingham, Dr. Cheeson, Dr. Blundean (Royal London Hospital, Whitechapel). I sincerely appreciate the advice of Vicky from the renal transplant clinic, about after care for renal transplant patients.

Also my thanks go to the Department of Social Services and Pensions, and the Housing Department. Most especially to Trevor Lawson at the Royal London Hospital, Whitechapel.

Also my uncle, Chief Tunji, Mrs. Kikelomo Oyelana, Mrs. Bunmi Omokeji (Mama B), Mr. Femi and Mrs. Jibola Aina, Mr. and Mrs. Johnson Owoyemi, Dr. Kola and Mrs. Funke Adebayo, Dr. Richard Omotoye, Dr. Akin Awofolaju, Dr. Soji Oladeinde, Mr. Tunji Talabi, Alhaji Yussuf, Alhaji and Alhaja Agbonmabiwon, Mr. and Mrs. Oshoba, Mama Gregg and Gregg, Blaise and Sarah Ekope, Euckay Ukandu, Mr. David and Mrs Shitu Oside, Mama Isale, Papa and Mama Median, Mama Helen Kambala, Mrs Ladipo, Otunba Yemi Taiwo, Dr. Adebisi, Paul

Adubi, Ayo Onatola, Idowu Oluyoye, Gbenga Owoseje, Akingbuyi Akintola, and Bolaji Adesanya.

I would also like to thank the following for their spiritual support: Dr. Abraham Chigbundu, Dr. Lawrence Tetteh, Dr. Ebenezer Tetteh, Pastor Tony Olufisan (crim), Pastor Bode Obasun, Papa Raphe and Mama Pitchou, Papa and Maman Amos (bxl) Papa and Maman Mokengo, Pasteur Tinos and wife. And everybody from the Spiritual Warfare Ministry, not only in London but all over the world.

I want to thank everybody that supported me during this agonising period.

Lastly I want to thank Joti Bryant, for her time and commitment in editing the book, and Alastair Chesson for his talented work on illustrations.

This book is dedicated to all renal (kidney) failure patients living, and those who have passed on, unable to live long enough to get a kidney transplant.

Chapter One

Understanding Kidney Function & Transplants

A normally functioning kidney separates urea, mineral salts and toxins that end up in the blood. The kidney filters the waste products and eliminates them from the blood. Secondly, the kidneys release hormones such as rennin, which helps to regulate salt levels, thereby regulating blood pressure. Thirdly, the kidneys conserve and monitor the body's balance of electrolytes, water and salts. Lastly, the kidneys regulate the calcium in blood for bone building, by producing an active form of vitamin D.

***

Kidney transplantation occurs when a donor's healthy kidney is placed into the body of a renal failure patient. The new kidney takes over the work of the failed kidney. Due to the unpredictable nature of kidneys available for transplant, statistics show that the number of people with kidney disease, needing transplants, continues to rise year after year. In Britain four years is the average waiting time for *cadaveric* kidney transplantation, unless a match is found immediately. Patients who receive *living* donor transplants have a shorter waiting time.

With chronic and end stage kidney failure, dialysis and kidney transplantation play a major role. When patients have suffered renal failure due to diabetes, hypertension, kidney disease, high cholesterol level and/or abusive use of over-the-counter medication, transplantation is an invaluable life-saving option.

There are situations whereby, due to liver disease, lung or heart disease, or a life threatening disease like cancer, or infections such as TB, kidney transplantation might not be considered. Another factor is when patients are very frail, or have a significant medical condition and the risk of transplantation failure may be too great. In these cases, it is less likely that kidney transplantation will be considered an option.

One of the main goals of successful kidney transplantation is to help patients to live a better quality of life and become more proactive. When you suffer from kidney failure you become a potential candidate for a kidney transplant. Whether or not to have, or to consider a transplant, depends on the benefits and disadvantages to the individual.

The main benefits of successful kidney transplantation are as follows:

. End of dialysis, giving more time.
. End to fluid restriction.
. A less restrictive diet.
. A possibility that women may bear children.
. Better quality of life.
. More energy.

Kidney transplants involve more than just the surgical procedure. A lot of issues have to be taken into consideration:

. Waiting several years before a match is found.
. The need to undergo surgery, with potential problems related to surgery and anaesthesia.
. Possibility that the transplanted kidney will be rejected, and ongoing dialysis reinstated.

. Taking anti-rejection pills for life.

. Conditions like hypertension or bone disease may worsen.

. Steroid medications recommended after kidney transplant have some long-term effects.

. Need to see doctors frequently at the transplant clinic, to ensure new kidney is functioning well.

. A bladder test may be needed, to see how the kidney is functioning.

Transplantation is not a total cure for kidney disease, but today the success rate has dramatically increased. It is worth noting that most live donors recover rapidly from the operation, and their long-term health is not usually affected by donating a kidney.

Matching donor organs to patients waiting for a transplant is based on a point system in the UK. Points are awarded for some of the following factors:

. How long a patient is on the waiting list.
. The level of the patient's antibodies.
. The donor's location.
. Donor tissue type and common antigens.

Note: Patients who are in the habit of not coming for dialysis, or skipping treatments, may find this affects their place on the list for a transplant.

The following vaccinations should be considered while waiting for a kidney transplant:

. Hepatitis B, highly recommended.
. Influenza — annually.
. Pneumonia — every five years.
. Diphtheria and tetanus — every ten years.

When evaluating a candidate for a kidney transplant, the consultant has to be sure that the transplant will be of benefit and safe for the patient, and also a match for the recipient. The following are some of the vital things taken into consideration prior to kidney transplantation:

BLOOD TYPE TESTING: A test is carried out to determine blood type, which falls into four inherited blood group types — A, B, AB, O. Notably, everyone fits into one of them. All patients for kidney transplantation must have their blood type confirmed before the operation, and the donor and recipient must have the same blood type, or be compatible.

HUMAN LEUKOCYTE ANTIGENS (HLA): Also called tissue typing. To carry out this test, blood samples from donor and patient are taken; no tissue is removed from the body. The test, which is performed on white blood cells, has special markers that reveal the tissue type inherited from parents.

VIRAL TESTING AND VIROLOGY: If you have been previously exposed to Hepatitis B, Cytomegalovirus (CMV), AIDS (acquired immune deficiency syndrome), and Epstein Barr virus (ERV), it is advisable you notify the transplant centre.

PANEL REDACTIVE ANTIBODY: This test shows the current state of the immune system. When the immune system is calm, it makes it easier for a prospective candidate to be operated on.

ANTIBODIES: Your body makes antibodies, which attack and fight off viruses and disease, but some antibodies attack the donor kidney, thereby causing irreparable damage, which kills the kidney.

CROSS-MATCHING: A cross-match test is done once a donor kidney is available. There are two types of cross-matching: compatible and incompatible. A compatible cross-match is when there is no reaction, a *negative* cross-match, whereas an incompatible cross-match is a *positive* cross-match, meaning that the kidney will not work. After the results and you are deemed fit for a transplant, this will enable the hospital to put you forward for the transplant list. Cross-matching is a very vital blood test. A final cross-match is done before the transplant.

TRANSPLANT WAITING LIST

In the United Kingdom, in order for you to have a transplant you must have been placed on the Transplant Waiting List. Your consultant will discuss with you the issues surrounding transplantation, and whether you have anyone capable of donating a kidney for you. If you suggest a family or friend, he/she will be evaluated for general health condition, and to see if the kidney is a match. You will then be put on a transplant list to receive a cadaveric donor kidney if the medical evaluation shows that you are a good candidate, without a family member or friend to donate for you.

Everyone on the waiting list in Britain is registered with the European centralized computer network, linking European countries. Some people wait several years for a good match while others wait within a few months.

It has been observed, that in the white population with kidney failure, generally the waiting time is shorter, as family or friends are more willing to donate for their loved ones. For the other ethnic groups like African, Afro-Caribbean and Asian, they wait longer, due to lack of donors from their particular group.

In kidney transplantation, the problem of ethics cannot be overlooked. There are people from the developing countries that do sell their kidneys probably due to poverty, while others are been coerced into parting with a kidney, due to financial difficulties. This is very sad indeed. See Part 1, Chapter 14, on donating a kidney to learn more.

It is very difficult living with kidney failure, due to the agony, frustration and complications associated with the sickness. This situation sometimes forces people to go and scout for kidney replacement in Third World countries.

Chapter Two

Preparing for my Kidney Transplant

The process of preparing for a kidney transplant started after I was diagnosed with kidney disease. I didn't know much about kidney failure. A friend of mine, while I was studying in Moscow in the former Soviet Union, told me he was left with only one kidney functioning, after a kidney was removed due to an infection. Whenever I saw him I was always full of pity for him, and I used to imagine how hard it must be to live with just one kidney, which to me was not a normal thing and seemed very strange.

Because of my curiousness after I was diagnosed with kidney failure, I asked my consultant what were my chances of surviving the sickness? He told me that I should not worry, that there are instances where people have, within six months of being on dialysis, received a kidney transplant. And that we should see how it goes. I might be lucky, and receive one within the next few months, or within a year. This was a consoling answer for me, as I was always thinking about death and total loss of everything.

On my second medical check-up, the results showed that I was not doing well with my dialysis. The doctor informed me that I needed changes to my treatment, and that I was also drinking a lot of fluid and the danger was that when the time of transplant came I might not be able to have a transplant, as my heart would be too weak to withstand the operation. I was advised to watch also my diet more carefully as I had high phosphate and potassium levels, and I was informed of the dangers involved with this. More questions were also asked about my medical history.

The third appointment was more focused on the transplant waiting list, as my results had improved, and I was asked if I had relatives that were ready to donate for me. After the meeting my wife discussed with me the possibility of donating. She volunteered to donate for me. I was actually delighted in the first instance, and then fear overcame me, as I was not well informed about the implications of donating an organ.

Most of the time I was sick I was always thinking about when death would come, and the total loss of everything. As she told me about wanting to donate a kidney to me, I became afraid; I thought if something compromised her own health as a result of donating kidneys, then the two of us were in trouble — there would be nobody to be around to take care of the children. I thanked her, but objected for this reason.

On my fourth check-up, I was informed there was an improvement in my blood results. Now my name had been put on the waiting list. A letter of confirmation of my name on the waiting list was sent to me on the 7th of May, 2004. In the letter I was advised of the following:

- Notify the transplant clinic of a change of address, or if travelling abroad.
- Inform the transplant clinic of a blood transfusion, or if pregnant.
- Ensure that the transplant nurse sends a blood test result for antibodies every three months.

The last time I was called for a transplant assessment, by Dr. Thuransingham, he informed me that he thought my time for a transplant was fast approaching, that I should continue the improvement on my dialysis, and keep my fingers crossed!

During that period, all the time I kept thinking about the day, the hour and minute that I would be telephoned, notifying me that I had a kidney donor.

Chapter Three

My Kidney Transplant

Notification of Kidney Transplant

Saturday, 5th July, 2008 around 01.00 a.m. I came home after my dialysis session and could not sleep. I was writing a letter of complaint about an incident that happened in the hospital, when a nurse was trying to decrease the amount of time I spent on the dialysis machine, from 4.5 hours to 4 hours. After finishing writing the letter, I typed and printed it out.It took me till 5.00 a.m. in the morning to finish the letter. I was tired and wanted to sleep, so I decided to lie down on the bed.

As I was still thinking how to get to sleep, I looked through the window; the sky was bright and clear. Not long after my mobile telephone rang, but I didn't get to it in time. I sat up to see who was calling me at that early morning at 05.26 a.m., thinking it was probably my mum calling from Nigeria; at times she calls me while going to the church for the early morning prayer, as she is a lay reader in her church, and at times prays for me there. I looked at my mobile phone and it did not show the caller's number. While I was still wondering who could have called me so early, the telephone rang again; it was now 05.36 a.m.

As I picked the phone up, I heard,
"Good morning. Can I speak to Adeleke Oyenusi."
"Speaking," I answered.
"Congratulations!"
"For what?" I asked.
"A kidney has been found for you."

I was silent. I could not express my joy and imagination, feeling still numbed and gobsmacked. It could not be a reality. It could not be true. It was like I was still dreaming. Could it really be true? After six years without a kidney, waiting on the transplant list for a suitable donor?

"Come straight away to the Royal London Hospital Whitechapel," the woman instructed.

I was in a panic, shaking and confused, not knowing what to do... This news... I could not contain myself.

Immediately, I woke the children up, the three of them came downstairs still half asleep, and could not understand why their dad had to wake them up so early, especially on a Saturday! When the children came downstairs, I said, "Congratulations." They were looking at each other, not understanding what was happening as none of their birthdays were due... Then I told them that their dad had been offered a kidney and I was going to the hospital straight away for a transplant operation. Then I told my eldest daughter to start the prayer for her dad, as their mother had gone to help a cousin who just lost her father and baby. The children were so delighted for me...

After I broke the news to them I burst into deep sobbing, I could not contain myself. Water started dripping from my eyes. The children could not contain my crying. I looked back at my life, the frustration, suffering, the anger and depression that followed my sickness for the past ten years. I could still not believe the news. It did not seem real to me in the first instance, but then all of a sudden the reality kicked in. What a moment of joy. What I had been waiting for years finally came to be.

I tried to reach my younger brother Albert Adeniyi Oyenusi, to break the news to him. He was not available. I phoned my other younger brother Pastor Femi Oyejobi. I reached his wife, Hassanah and I broke the news to her.

Then I looked at the letter, which I had carefully drafted, laughed and then said, "Devil. You are a liar." I read the letter once again, then I felt there was now no need to send the letter of complaint, and I tore the letter into pieces and threw it in the bin.

I booked a cab straight away and off I set for the hospital. On getting to the ward, I checked in still thinking about the message received early in the morning, reflecting on everything.

At about 10.30 a.m. I was called for a chest x-ray. A cross-match was done to check the compatibility with the donor kidney. This involved checking the blood, tissue typing and the kidney again. This normally takes about six hours to come back with the result. If the cross-match is negative, the transplant goes ahead, meaning there were no reactions, indicating there should not be a rejection.

Later, Dr. Zia, the Renal Department Registrar gave me the consent form to fill and sign and explained the operation procedure. He also explained the risks involved in the operation which are: bleeding, infection, delayed graft function, graft rejection, limping, and DVTPE (Deep Vein Thrombosis and Pulmonary Embolism). He later checked the veins in my groin and legs. Then Dr. Jacob Arlan came to check my lungs, heart and abdomen, and inserted a catheter in my right hand.

The renal nurse Adrian came to check my blood pressure which was 124/86, pulse which was 82, and oxygen saturation level which was also fine at 96. Then an ECG was performed to check the heart, and the result also was fine.

Before the result of the cross-match came I started to panic as I thought about what was happening, as I was earlier informed that the results would take only six hours. At about 6.00 p.m. the result of the cross-match came back, and the surgeon came to explain the procedure of the operation, what to expect during and after the operation. He informed me that the kidney was cadaveric (from a patient who died), and that the kidney does sometimes "sleep" for some time before it starts to function.

Once the blood started pumping round the kidney, this would eventually "wake up" the kidney, he explained. "If after the operation, the kidney doesn't start working or you don't pass urine in the early days for up to a week, do not get worried," he said. "The surgeon would have checked the kidneys and be convinced that it is going to work."

The anaesthetist came and explained the procedure under which the surgeon works with anaesthetic in the body. And that I would be injected with an anaesthetic ten minutes before the operation. It was explained that the kidney would be put inserted in the right groin. He informed me that the first 24 hours were crucial after the operation; after 24 hours I would be able to get out of bed and sit in a chair, and after 30 hours start walking around the ward.

Eventually the hour approached when I was to go to the theatre. In the ward the pain killer was given: PCA (Patient Control Anaesthetic), which lasts for five minutes. The nurse recommended pressing as many times as needed. I was the one in charge of my pain control. A catheter was inserted in a minor vein to measure the urine output, and could stay there for five days or longer. Another catheter was inserted to measure the central venous pressure and enable fluid intake. Also while in the ward oxygen was inserted into my nose. I was told this might make me thirsty afterwards, due to a lot of fluid being passed through me. I could also expect swelling on the feet, ankles and body.

I waited for the operation. At 10.45 p.m. on Saturday, 5th July, the time had come. My wife was with me and my bed was moved to the operating theatre. While I was entering the theatre, my wife and I held hands and we prayed together for God to allow everything to go well. I felt like crying, as I didn't know what fate I was to face. The entrance door to the theatre opened, my wife bid me well and the door closed again. I was injected with a high dose of anaesthetic and I was moved to the table with a gas mask on my face. That was all I remembered.

The operation finished around 4.00 a.m. in the morning. I was woken up after the operation and was later moved to my ward. I was very drowsy, and slept throughout the whole day. When I woke up a scan was done for me. Then I received a lot of telephone calls from friends and relatives, and well wishers.

I was informed that after the operation I would have to start to drink over five litres of fluid each day, so as to allow the kidneys to be wet and functioning, as for over four and a half years, I stopped passing urine. To drink five litres of fluid was unimaginable for me, as during my dialysis days, I was only allowed half a litre a day. After drinking so much I always felt like vomiting and my stomach was very heavy.

Monday, 7th July, 2008

I woke up feeling well. My blood pressure was alright at 119/92, oxygen level 95%, though my temperature was a bit high at 37.9. When my breakfast came, I tried to eat some cornflakes, but I soon became breathless, my body was collapsing and I felt like vomiting. I shouted to the nurse for help. After a time my condition stabilised and I fell asleep. The doctors later came to check me and an ultrasound was arranged. The result showed that the new kidney was fine. Later I went for dialysis for 2.5 hours. Only one litre of fluid was taken from me, due to the fact that the kidney was to be allowed more fluid so as not to become dry. A catheter was inserted into my private parts, to measure the urine production. I had only 30 ml but the surgeon told me not to worry, as my kidney was still "sleeping," and that it needed some time to adjust to my body.

Tuesday, 8th July, 2008

I woke up feeling extremely hot. I called for the nurse, who came to check my temperature. My temperature was extremely high: 39.8. The nurse called for the doctor, who came immediately to take a blood sample for analysis. The consultant was of the opinion that it might be the anti-rejection tablet that was the cause of my high temperature. I was only drinking water, as I was not hungry. Friends came to visit with get well messages. They all went home, and I was feeling bad again. My temperature soared again. I tried to sleep but could not. I was shivering and complained again to the doctors about the situation. They took my blood samples again to the laboratory. Later on I started to write my second book on my transplant experience.

Wednesday, 9th July, 2008

I woke up early with a high temperature. Antibiotics were prescribed for me. The porters arrived to take me for an ultrasound. The result showed an improvement in the kidney function. I went again for three hours of dialysis and three litres were taken out of me. After I felt so good and the breathlessness I was having stopped. I slept very well, just like a baby.

Thursday, 10th July, 2008
Woke up early about 05.20 a.m. Passed a little urine. Went to brush my teeth. I had not felt as good in myself for a long time — wonderful! I had a nice wash, and came back to the bedside. My nurse gave me an injection and came to change my wound dressing. Then I quickly felt like going outside for some fresh air. My nurse asked me to wait for lunch before going outside the building for fresh air. I could not wait to see the outside again. I quickly went to the Hanbury ward to say hello to the nurses and some other dialysis patients, and also said hello to Trevor Lawson, my Social Services worker, who was in the hospital.

Eventually I went out of the building to get some fresh air. Fantastic! Outside it was beautiful. The weather was bright; it was marvellous. But because of people smoking around me, I left the area and went to sit in the back garden of the hospital. I continued to wonder what had happened to me, how my new life would be adapted to. The fresh air was cool and breezy; I really enjoyed it.

The air was like that beside the ocean. After some time the rain started to fall and I had to go back inside. This was my first time out of the hospital, after four days. I was completely delighted to have progressed to this. My friends paid me another visit, and we all sat down in the guest room called the TV room to chat. After the visiting hour ended, I led them all to the main entrance of the building. They all left and I went back to my bed. I thanked the Lord to have reached this moment in my life. Then I slept, like a little new born baby.

Friday, 11th July, 2008

Woke up early, and used laxatives which made me jump to the toilet. I checked the time; it was 03.45 a.m. I took my urine bowl with me, as I was supposed to be noting the amounts of urine I passed each time and writing it down. Went back to my bedside, prayed and thanked the Lord. I was happy with the development of events. Asked for some ice cubes from my nurse. Started to write my manuscript again. After finishing, I shaved, thinking about my new life and the implications. Had my breakfast and took the required tablets. Went for dialysis very early and a total of 2.5 litres was removed from me. Came back for lunch and went again for ultrasound. Everything seemed alright. Came back and took my tablets, my neck line was removed, and had my antibiotics injection. Had supper with my wife. After we went to buy a TV card, and I led her to the exit. She left and I came back to the ward and slept.

Saturday, 12th July, 2008

Woke up early at about 02.50 a.m. Had to go to the toilet to empty my bowels due to the laxatives taken overnight. I took some urine samples, and went back to sleep. Woke up again and had my breakfast. Ran home to check my emails. Got a black cab home and back again. Doctors did the rounds, ward check. I was informed I had to go again for dialysis, in preparation for a biopsy on Monday morning. I went for dialysis and three litres were removed. After, some friends came to visit with my family. As they left, I fell asleep straightaway.

Sunday, 13th July, 2009

Woke up early at 03.45 a.m. Went to the toilet, slept again and woke up at 06.30 a.m. I felt good and started again writing my story. My tablets and injections taken. After lunch had some visitors. They left and I started thinking about the biopsy I was supposed to have the following day. Slept uncomfortably, as I kept thinking about the upcoming biopsy.

My Second Operation — Kidney Biopsy goes wrong

Monday, 14th July, 2008

Could not sleep well, as I thought about the biopsy operation: a long needle would be inserted from the outside of my stomach to the inside where the kidney is. (This would allow the doctor to remove small sections of the new kidney for examination, as the consultants keep on wondering why my new kidney was still sleeping.) Now waiting anxiously for the doctor to arrive. He later arrived and explained the procedure to me, but when I saw the long needle I got scared. The procedure started with the injection of pain killers to the site on my stomach. The doctor pressed the sharp needle inside my stomach; it was not very painful but I could feel something entering my body. The needle finally went in to my stomach and some of my kidney was extracted.

After the procedure was finished, I was told to lie down for the next six hours, though I lay down for ten hours. But I had a big problem after the procedure; I started to bleed a lot internally; I bled for over ten hours. While bleeding, I got concerned and agitated and kept on asking the nurses if I was going to bleed to death, as the blood refused to stop. The doctors got disturbed and asked for an ultrasound to be performed to see whether there was any internal damage. I was taken immediately for the ultrasound and the results showed no abnormality. Probably the reason was a small cut to a vein. The pain became so disturbing that I could not move out of bed. I just had to lie still. This was extremely difficult and inconvenient for me. But I had to do what had to be done. After some time I slept.

Tuesday, 15th July, 2008

Woke up and waited anxiously for the result of the biopsy. Had my breakfast and my prescribed tablets were given to me. The doctors did a ward visit. I hurriedly asked for the result of the biopsy. Looked straight into the eyes of the doctor as he told me that everything was fine, that I had to be patient to allow my body to get used to the new kidney, and that the kidney had not been rejected by my body. "The kidney is still sleeping," he replied, "keep your fingers crossed." I felt better when I heard this early morning news, I was so relieved. Later I was told that I would be going for dialysis. Took my tablets and injection and had my lunch. The porter came and I was taken for dialysis. The dialysis was for four hours with only one litre of water taken. Came back to the ward; several visitors, family and friends, were already waiting for me. Was desperately hungry, but fortunate as one of the nurses saved my dinner for me. Talked and chatted with my visitors; when it was time for the visitors to go they all left, and I went to bed early.

Wednesday, 16th July, 2008

Woke up early as usual. Had a shave and bath. Had my tablets and antibiotics injection given. Started to write my memoirs again.

My Third Operation

Thursday, 17th July, 2008

At about 4.00 a.m., I woke up with a terrible headache and a high temperature. I called for the nurse who I asked to check my temperature. My temperature had risen to 38.9 and while she was checking it, I fell asleep, wondering why my temperature was so high. All of a sudden, I noticed that my bed was wet, and I became so cold, wondering what might have happened.

I felt confused; I could not understand what was going on. Initially I thought this was a dream, as I thought it was impossible for me to wet the bed at this age. So I turned around on the bed to confirm my suspicions. I put on the bed light and looked at the bed, and saw my sheets full of dark red blood. I was scared and began to panic. I called the nurse, who later came to clean me up, and I asked her to immediately call for the doctor, so that he could have a proper look at me to confirm what was going on. She washed me and closed the curtains around me. I now began to bleed heavily.

When I sat down, the blood was just dripping, as if a water tap was turned on. So I decided to lie down flat on the bed, but still the same the blood would not stop for a second. I was confused, as I did not know what to do. I was expecting the nurse to quickly call for the doctor, but there was no response. The nurse was not even coming back to check on me, despite the fact that she knew I was bleeding heavily. The curtains were still closed around me. At about 5.20 a.m. I called my wife to come, as I felt I needed to see her before I finally died.

At 7.48 a.m., I heard the voice of a doctor I recognised, so I summoned the last ounce of energy in me, and stood up to call his attention to what was happening — that I needed immediate medical attention. As I stood up, with the last gasp in me and determination, he saw me, and our eyes were fixed on each other.

The whole floor was now full of blood. My attention was on explaining to him what I was experiencing. I tried to open my mouth, it was as heavy as a log, so I decided to move forward towards him, and I was now very near him. He now sensed something terrible was about to happen — I was about to fall down and collapse — so he moved quickly towards me. As I was still trying to talk,

I collapsed and fainted in his arms, as if he knew I was going to collapse. Dr. Gavin, a brave man, a man I respect and give honour to. A doctor that knows what to do at the most critical moment...

After I collapsed in his arms, I hardly knew what was going on. But I was later told that they put me back on the bed after Dr. Gavin had shouted to all the doctors and nurses to quickly come and help. (I cannot imagine falling on Dr. Gavin because I was a well built man, of over 90 kg.) Then they tried to resuscitate me.

Later on, I was already in the theatre for another operation, with a lot of nurses and surgeons at my side. In the theatre I was told about the procedure that was to take place and I was asked to sign the permission form, which I did. But I told them that before the procedure went ahead, I advised that an ultrasound should be done to see the position of things with my kidney. After the ultrasound it was clear that a vein that links to the kidney was cut and it was bleeding. So immediately they started the renal angiogram procedure.

It took over three hours to finish. After the doctor advised me that all the problems and defects had been resolved. Still confused but delighted to have witnessed another success, though still lying on the bed, I started to give glory and thanks to the Almighty, and I was thankful to the team that saved my life. I really appreciate the team's efforts in saving me, and bringing me back to life and joy. I really appreciate the work of the staff of the NHS, who do everything possible to preserve all our lives.

After the operation, I was brought back to the ward. I was asked what had happened by the nurses. I was of the opinion that there was negligence on the part of the nurse, the one who knew I was bleeding and never came back to see how I was doing, but shut the curtain around me. I bled for over two hours, unattended to... But I made them realise that I was just happy to be alive and that I did not want to make an issue of the situation, that they should just allow the situation to cool down and forget about the horrible experience. I was happy to carry on with my life without any complaints. But if this issue is used to improve the work ethic standard, that will be fine by me.

I was instructed to lie flat on the bed for eight hours without any movement so that the operation should settle down. I lay down the whole day, with pain all over my body, but it had to be done. My wife now by my side was so furious, angry and crying. She was consoled by the nurses and Dr. Gavin, Dr. Thurasingham and some other doctors. She was so annoyed; she wanted an issue made out of the case, but I asked her, "Aren't you happy to see me still alive?" So after a long conversation I asked her to drop the idea, and just be happy with the fact that I was alive. After some time I fell asleep. I did not know when she eventually left.

Friday, 18th July, 2008
I woke up around 4.30 a.m. and noticed stains on my body, so I went to the toilet to clean myself. Had my tablets and breakfast. I started to feel pain all over my body, headache, a temperature and high blood pressure. I thought it was normal after a big operation. My visitors came and they later left.

Saturday, 19th July, 2008

I woke up early, had my breakfast, and was called for dialysis. I went for four hours of dialysis and 3 litres were taken from me. My haemoglobin level went down to 6.3 due to the amount of blood I had lost during the last few days, so a blood transfusion was recommended for me. So I was given 4 bags of blood, long with antibiotics. After the dialysis I went back to my ward, and I felt so good in myself that I started to do my normal activities, which I could not do before. Had my lunch, and had a lot of visitors that day. They stayed with me for so long, over the visitors' recommended time. After they all left, I was extremely tired and I slept early.

My Fourth Operation

Sunday, 20th July, 2008

Woke up early as always, washed myself and had my breakfast. It was recommended that I go for ultrasound because my stomach got swollen and I could not stand up straight. I developed horrible pains in my stomach, so I called the nurses. Fortunately Professor Yakub was in the ward that Sunday morning, so I drew his attention to my plight. He had a thorough look at my stomach and wound site and felt me, and recommended that an ultrasound should be done immediately, without wasting any time. The porters came and took me straightaway for an ultrasound. They detected some abnormalities in my stomach. The result was sent to my doctor, who informed me that an immediate operation had to be performed, to remove the abnormalities in my stomach. I was devastated; I couldn't understand the fate that had befallen me. It was like one step forward and two backwards. This caused me to have a lot of thought about my life. This problem became a big concern for me. In this process of thinking about this problem my younger

23

brother arrived and comforted me, told me not to worry too much about the problem.

I was told not to eat or drink until after the operation, in the evening.

My wife also came and I explained the situation to her and she also was highly positive about the whole affair and supportive, and quoted the bible: "What God has done, he has already done it." She told me that I should not worry, or be afraid, and that it was for the glory of God. All the time I kept on thinking about the whole episode. I was waiting anxiously to be taken to the theatre. My younger brother went back to St. Albans, and I was left with Gisele and my son Kenneth. Waited for the porter to take me to the theatre.

The porter came for me around 21.45 p.m. and I was feeling fine again, until 22.15 p.m. when I was put to sleep for my operation. They woke me up around 2.00 a.m. and brought me back to the ward. The blood and water clot in my abdomen and the one surrounding the kidney were successfully removed, and all properly cleaned and sewn back up. A short time after coming back to my ward, I was fast asleep.

Monday, 21st July, 2008

Woke up, feeling extremely well in myself. Phoned my wife early in the morning, to tell her that everything went well and that I was now feeling alright, compared to the other day before the operation when I could not stand up from the bed. I had my tablets and breakfast. I was still not very stable and was advised to stay in bed for the whole day. I was again thinking about the fate that had befallen me with all this operation. Overall I was very optimistic and determined. I had to accept that what was happening in my life was real and genuine. Visitors came and left and I slept.

Tuesday, 22nd July, 2008

Woke up and had my breakfast. The doctor made a ward inspection. I was to go for dialysis in the morning, which was later changed to the afternoon. Had my lunch and about 14.00 p.m. and the porter came to take me for my session. After the dialysis, I felt good in myself and was brought back to the ward. I started to walk and felt lighter in myself. Had my dinner, with a lot of visitors waiting for me. We chatted for a long time. After they left, I went to my bedside, started to write my memoirs. Then fell asleep.

Wednesday, 23rd July, 2008

Woke up feeling great in myself. Had my breakfast and the doctors came round. Impressed with my progress. I was informed that my phosphate level was high; it went to 2.7 mmol/L. Told about the possibility of new medication: changing phosphate binders from Calci-chew to Phosex and Renagel, which I used to take before my transplant operation. They advised that we just take things one at a time, after I complained too much about the fact that my kidney was still sleeping.

Another Biopsy Scheduled

Thursday, 24th July, 2008

Woke up and had my breakfast. Washed myself. The doctors came for a ward check. One of the doctors came to have a chat with me about possibility of another biopsy, as they wanted to know if my body was trying to reject the kidney. He could not figure out why the kidney was still not functioning as expected. He was of the opinion that if something was to go wrong they could quickly sort the problem out early, to avoid any complications. After hearing this news I was totally devastated, because of my previous experience with the biopsy procedure.

All my hopes and aspirations disappeared within seconds. He went to tell me that my situation was unique, as only one in hundred had the kind of complications I had. He wanted to be sure that I was not having a rejection, as it would be dangerous not to start to treat the kidney if it was to reject, as this could cause the kidney to completely die, or incapacitate me. The sorrow in my head was immeasurable, after already going through this life-threatening operation.

I was shivering and scared to death, because all my complications came from the biopsy. A lot of questions came to dominate my thoughts about the next step to take. I became confused. I did not know which way to go forward — to go on with the second biopsy, or allow the kidney to reject totally. I was frustrated. But the doctors had to do what was needed to be done. I am a lay man as far as medicine is concerned. The fact was that they were not satisfied with the results they were getting from my kidney, which after three weeks was not working and still sleeping. I sobbed and cried a lot as I could not understand why my life had to be as hard as this, with so many disappointments. I was devastated, but not destroyed, bent but not cracked.

I phoned my wife and told her about the situation. She asked that we pray, which we did, and we left it at that. But I was thinking what fate I was having in my life. Life had been so unfair to me. What had I done to be rewarded this way? Total devastation. After talking to the doctor we agreed that the biopsy should not be immediate and that on Monday, we should have a look at how things were. If the index got better, then there would be no need for another biopsy, but if things stayed the same, then they should carry out the biopsy on Monday. So we all agreed on this. But I was scared to death, after four consecutive operations in less than 15 days. Now I was expecting the fifth operation; this was ridiculous. I could not believe what was happening. This could not be true.

As I was still thinking about what I was hearing from the doctor, there was a ward check. The junior doctors were of the opinion that things were a bit better and improving, and that with my kidney I just had to be patient before everything started to go well. This gave me a bit of comfort. Later Dr. Mark Blundean came and told me that he understood my fears and concerns and that he would come on Monday to come and take charge of the biopsy himself. "Don't worry, everything will be alright," he said to me. "I will come at eight a.m. to do the operation myself." The nurse came to do my weight. She happened to be a Nigerian, Mrs. Kupoluyi, and she advised me at length about the situation, and comforted me. She then removed the catheter from my stomach.

Had my lunch and another of my younger brothers Pastor Femi Oyejobi, with Hasanah his wife came and prayed with me. He gave me the confidence and support which I needed. Dr. Junaid and Dr. Kulsoom Junejo came to see me. They had a chat with me and left. My visitors came and left and because my mind was disturbed, I went to bed immediately after they went.

Friday, 25th July, 2008
Woke up early around 4.30 a.m. in the morning and went to the toilet. Stayed a long time, and then went back to the ward. Had a sharp pain in my back and heart. This was the beginning of something horrible. I was in total pain and agony. It was as if my heart was about to explode. I shouted for the doctor, who came and I explained my situation to her. The nurse came and measured my blood pressure which was 200/90. My temperature also went up drastically. Oxygen was put in my nose to ease my diminished breathing. Immediately an ECG was

performed on me. It was normal, but the pain in my heart and back would not ease.

I wanted to call my wife, but was not allowed to do that as I was in a terrible state, and was not to cause more panic. But when things had improved for me around 5.30 a.m. I was allowed to call her and I explained to her about my ordeal. She was in a panicky situation and was already on her way to the hospital. I fell asleep after talking to her. I opened my eyes to see her sitting by my side. I began to tell her what had happened.

A friend of mine, Mr. David Shitu Oside was also called for a transplant operation. He had visited me earlier and had told me that he was the next on the list for a transplant. He came to break the news of his admittance to the ward for his transplant, but I was fast asleep. By the time he came the second time I had woken up. He broke the news to me that he had been called in the morning to go to the hospital. I was so delighted for him. He left for dialysis in preparation for his operation. I could still not understand what had happened to me in the early morning. My wife was consoling me, as I felt extremely disturbed. The doctors came around and I explained what had happened, and the ordeal I faced with the heart pain and back pain.

My New Kidney Functioning

I showed the doctors the amount of urine I had collected. They were happy and delighted at the amount; they even clapped for me and for my success. It was encouraging. For the first time I could actually see an improvement in my urine production. They were of the opinion that if the urine increased and other levels also improved, then there would be no need for the biopsy on Monday. They left the ward feeling delighted for me. Throughout the day I was over the moon about this great news, which kept lingering in my mind. Although I thought the kidney had finally kicked in and the possibility of another biopsy was fading hour by hour, I still could not forget the first experience I had with a biopsy. My wife came later and I divulged the good news to her. She was also very happy and delighted for me. I slept through the night like a new born baby. My urine collection for the day was 450 ml.

Saturday, 26th July, 2008
Had my tablets, shaved, washed and dressed. Feeling great, and calm. My younger brother came in the morning to see how I was doing. Later I decided to go home and pick up my computer because I had some outstanding jobs to complete for my book, and I wanted to check my emails. It had been about one month since I left the house. So I had my lunch and booked a cab to set for the journey, but while in the cab my condition changed. I felt sweaty and felt like vomiting. I developed a horrible headache and my situation got worse. I started to vomit. I opened the passenger window and my head was now stuck out of the car and I started to vomit terribly. This did not cease, and the taxi driver had to stop constantly on the way to the house.

We reached the house, I checked my letters, packed the computer and we immediately left again for the hospital. My situation became frightening, stopping the cab every five minutes, but in the end we arrived back in the hospital. I was happy that we came back to the hospital. My brother was so annoyed with me for the unwarranted risk which I took. I could see the anger, frustration and disturbance in his eyes, as he asked what if something had happened on the road? I did agree with him that it was an error of judgement, and told him I was sorry.

By now I was bored with the hospital environment; I needed something to do, to keep my body and soul together, in the form of an activity, which I thought having my computer would help me with. I felt so bad and ashamed of myself for putting my younger brother through this kind of ordeal. I called the nurses to do an ECG, to measure my blood pressure and oxygen level. After some time my blood pressure stabilised. My younger brother left and I went to sleep, thinking about my ordeal. On Saturday my urine collection measured 750 ml.

Sunday, 27th July, 2008

Woke up early at about 4.30 a.m. and went to the toilet. I started to feel uneasy, and felt a terrible pain in my back. This was the kind of sharp pain which I normally felt when my blood pressure was high. In my heart I was feeling another terrible pain, as if an arrow was piercing through my heart and lungs. I started to shout for the nurse, who rushed in to see me in terrible pain. I immediately asked her to check my blood pressure and my oxygen level, and to perform an ECG.

My blood pressure had soared and I asked that I should be given a blood pressure tablet to lower my blood pressure. For ten years I had been suffering with high blood pressure and when I was in this situation, I normally dashed for my blood pressure tablets, which bring the blood pressure under control. I started to shout because I was in total pain and agony, even lashing at the poor gentle lady doctor, just doing her job the way she deemed fit. The nurses had to do the ECG and other things before the doctor could prescribe medication, but I was in pain and shouting that I be given the blood pressure tablets immediately. You could understand my situation, and I could also understand the doctor's position as she could only prescribe after full confirmation of the current test results.

After the results I was given Amlodopine 10 mg and the pain started to ease. I was also given Nitro lingual under the tongue to help ease the pain. After some time the pain eventually eased and I had to tell the doctor and the nurse treating me that I was extremely sorry for my actions and that I did regret it. They all accepted my apology, and this gave me some idea of what the NHS staff have to cope with while doing their jobs. The pain ceased finally and I slept with the oxygen tube in my nose.

After I woke up, I was now strong enough to start the final corrections on part 2 of my book. This I did till lunch time. Finished with my lunch and started the corrections again, as I was determined to finish corrections on the book that same day.

Told that I needed a blood transfusion. I waited for the doctor to put on the line on my hand. Informed that I would be given two packets of blood, due to my haemoglobin level dropping. I finished with the blood transfusion, had my evening tablets, and started to jog my memory about the events of the past week so that I could put them into writing. My urine collection for Sunday was 1200 ml from 8.00 a.m. to 12.00 p.m.

Monday, 28th July, 2008

Woke up late because I went to sleep late, thinking about what I would be faced with after the doctor's announcement today. Had my breakfast. The nurses took my blood pressure, oxygen level and checked my weight. Now waiting for the doctors to arrive. In a panicky situation over the announcement about my kidney biopsy. My mind was confused... The news I did not want to hear was that the biopsy will go ahead. This will not happen, I kept saying, and praying within myself. I was very concerned.

Eventually the moment came, when the doctors approached and I was looking straight into their eyes, ready to hear them tell me about the biopsy. They looked straight into my eyes and the conversation that followed was, "For the past two days, we looked at your urine collection and the result of the blood sample. The creatine level has decreased and the urea level has also decreased. We are impressed, and there will not be any need for another biopsy." I opened my mouth wide with surprise, as this was not the news I was expecting. I was waiting for something negative and here I was with a positive result.

The joy in me was immeasurable as I opened my mouth wider. And could not close it. That moment, the joy was something else. I did not want another biopsy after my first experience. It was stressful thinking about the first biopsy. I was delighted with myself and the doctors. Then I was left to think about the early morning news and the impact of this news on my life. I was also informed that if things continued the way they were going, I might be discharged in two days time.

This also brought great joy to me as I was very fed up with the hospital environment, and was over the moon with the news, this new reality. The doctors left, and the pharmacist came to inform me that she now had to teach me how to manage with my medications when I was discharged. She explained everything to me and she left.

Had my lunch, and slept. My wife came and I explained the whole situation to her. She was delighted for me. She stayed with me and I decided that we have a stroll, to exercise my legs and muscles as I did not get out of bed for many days. My walking had improved slightly but I was still struggling with my balance. She stayed with me for a long time. We talked about everything, about outstanding problems, and that this was the time to review our matrimonial issues. She left and I started writing again in my manuscript, and in the process fell asleep.

Tuesday, 29th July, 2008

Woke up and had my breakfast. I went to the toilet and I noticed a lot of blood in my urine; this was very frightening and disturbing and I started to panic, shaking. I heard the voice of the doctor and hurried to see him and told him about what was happening. He told me it was normal for a new transplanted patient to have blood in their urine. This could be as a result of the stent that connects the bladder to the kidney. He then sent a sample of the urine to the laboratory. Do not worry, he told me. I was so relieved to hear his words. I then started to pray after this news, for God's total support. The doctors did a ward check and were delighted with my blood results. There was a big increase in my urine production, within twenty four hours, I had already produced 1.81 litres of urine and my creatine level dropped dramatically, to 120 points, which was very interesting to the doctors.

Had my lunch, my wife and my younger brother Pastor Femi Oyejobi visited me. They prayed with me and exchanged views on religious matters. The blood continued to appear in my urine, the whole day. My wife and brother eventually left. I do not remember when I fell asleep.

Wednesday 30th July, 2008

I was now very fed up with the hospital; I was home-sick. I woke up around 2.00 a.m.; I could not stand the hospital environment any longer. When it was 5.00 a.m. I booked a taxi and off I set for the house. On arrival I knocked the door for my wife to open. She was surprised to find me standing in front of the house. "Leke how you can do this?" she said. She opened the door and we went upstairs and chatted for some time and off I went, back to the hospital.

Preparing for Final Discharge from the Renal Ward

Had my breakfast and waited for the doctors' ward inspection. They confirmed to me that I had a massive improvement and that if the early morning results were good I might be allowed to go home that same day. I could not believe this early morning news. It was a shock, as I earlier thought I would still be in the hospital for another week. I could not contain my happiness, it was beyond me. I was happy and delighted with myself. I immediately phoned my wife to break the news to her. She was extremely happy for me.

Had my lunch, then there was the ward inspection, with the nurses and doctors. The consultant also repeated to me that the results were good and that I was allowed to go home but I still had to go through the procedure of learning how to manage with my tablets. I had to stay the night, to get accustomed to the procedure. I was a bit devastated, as I really wanted to go home. But I thanked the Lord, to have witnessed this entire event. I had to wait for the doctor's instructions. After my visitors left, I was left alone, to start counting the minutes and hours before finally going home.

Thursday 31st July, 2008
Woke up at about 5.00 p.m. with the excitement of finally going home filling my head. I could not wait any more minutes. I just wanted to get out of the hospital. The joy of going back home to my family was immeasurable. I wanted to jump inside the car and instantly be back home. The joy, and happiness, knowing that all my problems were behind me, made me sob and cry. My eyes

were red like burning fire. I just could not contain myself and my emotions.

Can you imagine it? I was like a prisoner let loose. What a moment of joy! Now I could be a happy man again. The feelings are too hard to explain. Can you imagine the mood of a young boy, after being given an ice cream? The laughter in my eyes could be seen. A friend Bola, (who was working at the hospital when I was admitted for kidney failure in 2002), saw me and said, "Everything in you has changed. You look like a new born baby. Your talking, your laughter. And I can now see the handsome face of yours again."

The staff nurse came to insert a catheter into my hand for an infusion, so I implored her to start the procedure straight away so that it could be finished early. She agreed and went to prepare the solution and the procedure started, and during the process I continued with my book writing.

The procedure finished, my medications were prepared for me and now I was just waiting for the discharge letter. They gave me the discharge letter, and then I was waiting for my wife to pick me up, before I could say goodbye and thank you for the care and marvellous work of the staff at Pauline ward of the Royal London Hospital, Whitechapel. (It was a marvellous experience. This you have to live through yourself, to be able to appreciate the good work, the pressures and tolerance, dedication and intelligence of the NHS staff. You cannot feel it from outside; you need to be there in order to appreciate them.)

It was difficult for me on the one hand to leave these marvellous people, but on the other hand I was just happy to have gone through the ordeal and survived. I missed my family; my wife and children. My wife came, we bid goodbye to everybody and departed for the house. On getting to the house everything looked different after a month's absence. I was extremely tired and dashed to the bedroom and slept like a new born baby. I cannot remember the last time I slept so deeply; snoring terribly, I was told later by my children. Anyway, they could understand.

The following day I praised the Lord for a good ending to my ordeal. I rang to tell some of my friends that did not know that I had been discharged, as they continued to go and pay me a visit in the hospital. I started to receive phone calls of congratulations. A lot of people were joyful and glad for me. Some prayed and also wished me well.

I had to drink a lot of water, about three litres per day, to allow the kidney to continue to function properly. I started to urinate every five minutes. This was not convenient for me as I had to be going for the toilet each time. To me this was not normal, as over four and half years I had not been urinating. I could not hold my bladder. I had to have a bottle by my side as the urine could come any time. Another thing of joy for me was the stoppage of blood in my urine after leaving the hospital. I started to take my tablets as stipulated, as I was warned about the dangers I might face if I did not.

In the house, there was a total change. The environment improved. I am now a very quiet person, reserved and born again. The love I have for my family is great; I wish I could travel all over the world with them, to compensate them for the lost ten years. With my sickness, they had to put up with a lot most, especially the anger, frustration of my sickness and my depression.

Only God that can compensate the children, especially at their tender age, to have witnessed all the bad moments of my sickness. I hope when they grow up, they will be able to understand that life is full of ups and downs, and that no condition is permanent. I hope my sickness will make them stronger in life and help them to be ready for any eventuality in life.

I BLESS THE LORD FOR THEM.

Chapter Four

Attitudes, Beliefs, Faith, Spirituality & Religion

This chapter is meant to be a continuation of chapter 12, part 1 of my book, *Living a Normal and Healthy Life After Renal (Kidney) Failure.* (It is recommended that you get a copy of part 1 of my book, so as to understand my views on attitudes and religion.) This chapter places emphasis not only on medical science but also on the spiritual role of prayers in the healing process. Religion should be part of an integral part of our healing process. Actually, nearly everybody prays when faced with life threatening illness, or for any debilitating disease or condition.

Nowadays prayers are being used as an integral part of healing. Many people now want treatment from the mind, body, soul and spiritual perspective. Additionally, many scientists feel that science and spirituality enhance each other and do not represent incompatible views of the world. One of them is Albert Einstein, who stated that: "Science without religion is lame and that religion without science is blind." (1)

As I said earlier, I don't want to pick arguments on this issue but to offer my point of view, give my own advice on this subject matter and to contribute to this delicate area of thinking. We — especially from the ethnic minority groups, Africans, Afro-Caribbean and Asians — have to re-examine our belief structures and the way we perceive issues, when it comes to religion and our health. I believe I am not alone in my way of thinking. We have to be able to engage constructively and criticise what we believe is not right and might be of danger to our life.

I do not support the Christian way of extortion, coupled with misinformation and misinterpretation which is practised in some religious quarters nowadays.

Another thing worth mentioning is that some Christian brothers and sisters have abandoned their loved ones, in the name of serving God. Here they have misinterpreted the scriptures. They are not serving God, because Jesus Christ is love.

My views and beliefs remain the same on this matter. That is, do the right thing by going to the hospital to find out what your health concerns are, and then back yourself with your prayer. I highlighted the dangers one might face by confusing religious beliefs with medical treatment.

Please note that health problems are extremely serious with kidney failure, and that you cannot put sentiment before your medical treatment. You may die if you put sentiment before treatment.

If you are sick with kidney failure, the best place to be is in the hospital for you to be properly looked after, not to start sleeping in the churches, mosques or the traditional healers' houses. Your condition requires urgent medical support and attention. Then back yourself up with your prayers.

As I said in part 1, God is very capable but you need to be realistic about your condition and the situation at hand. The ignorance associated can have catastrophic effects. If you are sick, go to a medical doctor, one that is well trained, and qualified to take care of your specific medical condition.

As for me, I combined the wisdom of medical science and innovation with the power of the Almighty, and the combination worked for me. I believe in the healing power of prayer, that is why before I go for my dialysis I visit the church to pray for God's intervention on my behalf concerning my health issues. God will do it for me, but I put effort into playing my own part in the healing process. There is a role for medical science, likewise prayers. What I am trying to say is that we should use our prayers wisely, and not be dogmatic about our religious beliefs.

Religion with prayers, and medical science, complement each other. Heaven helps those who help themselves. (2). Prayer does help by fortifying you, that is fortify your belief structure. It makes you strong in times of despair, and helps restore your confidence.

There were times, when I thought everything was over for me, but I have sailed through the health difficulties with the help of the Almighty. In the Bible in the Book of Psalms chapter 30, verse 5, (3) it says: "Weeping may endure for a night but joy cometh in the morning."

There were situations when I got confused in my life with my sickness, but I had the belief that God would find a way for me and I would sail through. In the Bible in the Book of Joel, chapter 2 verses 23 – 30, (4) he talks of the mercy and restoration of God.

There were situations that I was spiritually down, waking up in the middle of the night, crying, dejected but I got my consolation from the Almighty.

I had bid myself good-bye before I slept and I felt I would never wake the following day, but I woke up the following morning feeling good and happy. These instances were many, and I have managed to bounce back. It took ten years of constant prayers before my prayer manifested. With God you cannot be in a hurry. The way God does his work is inexplicable.

In the Bible in the Book of Psalms 62, verse 11 – 12, (5) he says: "Power and mercy belong to me." God has spoken once. Twice I have heard this. That power belongs to God, also to you, Oh lord of mercy. I had the belief that God would do it for me. In the Bible in the Book of Habakkuk chapter 2, verse 3, (6) it states that the time he has set aside will surely come. He has the time for everything. "For the nation is yet for an anointed time. But at the end it will speak and it will not lie. Though it tarries wait for it. Because it will surely come. It will not tarry."

Though it was a gruesome and cruel journey during my sickness, I can confirm the hand and glory of God in my life. God was merciful to me. I am blessed and I give honour and glory to God, to be able sit down today and put all these events in writing.

As I said earlier, I don't want to be associated with practising Christianity that discourages sick patients from seeking medical attention when they are really in need of it. Our prayer should be used as an instrument and weapon to strengthen ourselves; it should not be a blockage to our general well-being.

Let us give honour to whom honour is due, and respect to whom respect is due. Don't let us play the role of the Almighty. We should not underestimate the significance and role of the doctors, surgeons, and nurses and what they are doing in helping us with our health concerns. So also the role of prayers in our lives. Both have a role to play in our lives. We should know that God giveth the doctors, surgeons and nurses the wisdom and vision to take care of our health problems. We have to be realistic about our prayers and not to be dogmatic.

I had to change the pattern of my prayer when I was praying for God to jump start my kidney again, while I was waiting to go for an operation for Continuous Ambulatory Peritoneal Dialysis (CAPD). Initially my prayer stated that my body is the temple of Christ, and no knife should cut me open. I eventually changed the wording of my prayer for the CAPD operation, to let God allow the operation to be successful without any preconditions, and that the operation serve the purpose for which it was meant. My prayer changed and the operation went successfully. With God you cannot dictate to, and you cannot be in a hurry.

Another example was when I had the feeling that I would have a transplant operation in 2004; the year went by and I was not called for a transplant operation; the following year came and again I was still not called. So the following year I changed the wording of my prayer to: "God I am no longer in a hurry, but bless me with a functioning kidney transplant at your own chosen time. Give me a kidney that will make me glorify and elevate your name." After two years of changing the wording of my prayer, I was called for a kidney transplant. I glorify his name; I was the only one on the waiting list suited for that particular kidney. Often there are situations whereby two, three or four patients will be vying for the same kidney, due to the shortages in kidney donors. Let the name of the Lord be glorified. Amen.

With my sickness the devil planned total destruction for me, but God helped me sail through, made me stronger, and prepared marvellous things for me in my life. The day I had my transplant operation was the beginning of my salvation and healing process. I cannot describe the pain and agony I went through; I went to heaven and back, but I was not consumed by the fire of the devil. God dwells in me; he showed me his compassion and mercy. God opened me up to learn more about life, through the frustration and challenges of my sickness, but he consoled me at last with a blessing of a new kidney. He made me stronger for the problems and challenges of life.

I had been lonely and cried at times, with painful and sorrowful cries, but God showed me his faithfulness and mercy. I will sing Hosanna, and praise his name and the blessings of the Lord... I read Psalm 23: "The Lord is my shepherd, I shall not want..." (7) The Lord made me have my victory at last. Psalm 121: "I lift up my eyes to the hills. From whence comes my help. My help comes from the Lord who made heaven and earth..." (8) Psalm 123: "Unto you I lift my eyes. O you who dwell in the heavens..." (9) The Lord is omnipotent and merciful. God will not allow destruction in our life. That is why I will continue to give honour and glory to the Lord, who has stretched his hand of healing into my life.

Have the endurance and patience so that the Almighty can manifest in your life. My situation and condition bent me, but I was not broken; God made me sail through without death. With my sickness, I have always prayed for the lord to give me the strength to be able to battle through and be strong again. I am a victor, a living example of God taken action in people's lives. God's promises never failed in my life.

I pray with you at this moment, to help you remember that whatever you might be going through with your health condition, the Lord is your strength and salvation, and he will surely make a way for you to sail through. Ask for God's guidance and mercy.

In the next paragraph, I highlight the instances when my prayer, and divine intervention, saved me from death. This is divided into two parts: before my transplant and during my transplant process.

- Unable to sleep at night, I forced myself to go and check out what my health problems were, as I was having uncontrollable, high blood pressure. I thank the Lord that I went to the hospital that day; I could have dropped dead from high blood pressure.
- Fell down with a stroke. My wife and son were praying hard for my recovery. I believe the Lord looked at my little son and granted me life again.
- Diagnosed as potentially developing Multiple Sclerosis. The second day it turned out not to be the terrible nightmare I was expecting.
- Started to use my legs to work after the stroke. How I witnessed this moment in my life.
- Overcame the problem of my stroke. How I recovered fully, and how God turned my sorrow into joy and happiness.
- The day I became breathless, thinking I was going to go and die in the hospital, it was detected my kidneys were no longer functioning.
- My prayers and dreams convinced me to change my prayer, to have my transplant operation.
- Lucky to be alive after my CAPD infection.
- Hospital bed found for me. I developed an infection called Peritonitis, after seven days without receiving proper treatment. With prayers on that faithful Sunday, I was offered a bed at my regular hospital.
- Problem of haemodialysis. How I was able to sail through it: I locked myself in my room and prayed vehemently for God's intervention to save me.
- Overcoming the problem of over drinking fluid. More than my recommended half a litre a day, which could have led to my heart collapsing. Prayer led to my determination to succeed with my treatment.

Instances before/after my transplant where God took action and showed me mercy

- I was miraculously called for a kidney transplant, after an incident that forced me to write a letter of complaint about a nurse that was bent on reducing my time on the dialysis machine from 4.5 hours to 4 hours. I used my inner thoughts to destroy the letter of complaint.
- The news of my transplant operation was broken to me.
- When my bed was moved to the operating theatre I prayed with my wife that the operation be successful. The operation was successful.
- Biopsy went wrong with terrible consequences, with the blood failing to stop.
- Nurse closed the curtain on me and I was left bleeding. I lost a lot of blood, leading to another operation being performed on me. The operation was successful.
- Proposal of another biopsy for Friday, 25th July, 2008 and things turned around for me on Saturday when my kidney jump-started. The first day I started to urinate after over four years of not being able to urinate.
- Problems I had while I went to pick up my computer from the house, when my physical condition got worse.

I believe that the Lord takes control and brings about changes in our lives. I had the belief that God would make me sail through everything, and being able to live through ten years of sickness shows the hand and mercy of the Almighty, and the glory of God in my life.

"With God no hope is lost, and all things are possible."- Matthew, chapter 9, verse 26.

When you are down spiritually, take your Bible and read it. Use the power of your prayer to strengthen your faith, and comfort yourself.

The following Bible passages are some of those I used to console and comfort myself. They made me stronger, fortified my belief, while I battled for healing, helped me to forge ahead and restored my confidence. While I was doing the right thing, for example for the six years I had the kidney failure, I never once missed a dialysis session, I always used the following Bible passages to back myself up.

- Deuteronomy 7, verse 15. "And the Lord will take away from you all sickness and will affect you with none of the terrible disease of Egypt which you have known but will lay them on all those who hate you."(10)
- Psalms 6, verse 2. "Be merciful to me Lord, for I am faint; oh Lord heal me for my bones are in agony."(11)
- Psalms 91, verse 9-10. "Because thou hast made the Lord which is my refuge, even the most high thy habitation. There shall no evil befall thee neither shall any plague come near thy dwelling."(12)
- Isaiah 41, verse 10. "So do not fear, for I am with you, do not be dismayed for I am your God, I will strengthen you and help you. I will uphold you with my righteous right hand." (13)
- Isaiah 54, verse 17. "No weapon formed against you shall prosper and every tongue which raises against you in judgement you shall condemn. This is the heritage of the servants of the lord and this righteousness is from you says the lord." (14)
- Jeremiah 17, verse 14. "Heal me O Lord and I shall be healed, save me and I shall be saved, for thou art my praise." (15)

- Jeremiah 33, verse 6. "Behold I will bring you health and healing. I will heal thee and reveal to them the abundance of peace and truth." (16)
- Matthew 7, verse 7-8. "Ask and it shall be given to you seek and you will find, knock and it will be opened to you. For everyone who asks receive and he who seeks finds and to him who knocks it will be opened." (17)
- Matthew 21, verse 22. "Whatever you ask in prayer with faith, you will receive." (18)
- Mark 11, verse 24. "Therefore I say whatsoever things you ask when you pray, believe that you receive them and you will have them." (19)
- Luke 10, verse 19. "Behold, I give you unto you power to thread on serpents and scorpions and over all the power of the enemy and nothing shall by no means hurt you." (20)
- Romans 8, verse 11. "But if the spirit of him who raised Jesus from the dead dwells in you. He who raised Christ from the dead will also give life to your mortal does through his spirit who dwells in you." (21)
- John 5, verse 14 – 15. "Now this is the confidence that we have in him that we ask anything according to his will, he hear us, whatever we ask we know that we have asked of him." (22)

My prayers were centred on the following aspects:
- God's healing power.
- God's mercy on my life.
- God's grace in my life.
- God's anointment in my life.
- God's comfort in my life.

The steps I took in my prayers:
- I first ask for the Lord's forgiveness in my life.
- I open my heart to the Lord.

- I praise his name.
- I ask for my heart's desire.
- I also remember in prayer other people in need like me.

An example of a PRAYER FOR FORGIVENESS:

Lord Jesus Christ, I solemnly ask for the forgiveness of my sins. Please give me the power and strength to forgive. You have shown me mercy in the past and you continue to show me mercy. Purify my heart and mind today, with the belief that you have forgiven me. I thank you for your grace at this moment. Lord I do solemnly and honestly forgive everybody that has harmed me. I do pray at this moment for the grace and spirit of forgiveness. I bless your name and thank you that I am freed from the evil of unforgiveness. Let your holy spirit light me up and enlighten every dark area of my mind. Amen.

In times of despair or disturbance, the following prayers can be consoling. It is good to be persistent with prayers for healing. Be specific with your prayers, especially issues connected to your illness. Ask the Lord to change your negatives into positives, and finally don't allow despair to get the upper hand in your life. Have the belief that when you are praying, the Lord is where you are right at that moment.

Oh Lord, I cover myself with the blood of Jesus. You are my protector. I surrender myself completely to you. Satan I command you in the name of the Lord Jesus Christ to leave me, with your demons. Heavenly father I am thankful for the armour and protection you have provided. I claim victory in my life. I reject all satanic temptations in my life. Look upon me with the power of mercy. Comfort me and give me patience during my affliction. Oh Almighty, I call on you for total healing and for the grace of God.

God, visit me in time of need, relieve thy sick servant from the pain and agony; have mercy on me, and give me the patience to cope with this sickness. God, restore my stolen health. God, in your mercy, uproot every evil spirit planted in my body working against me and my body. May you come and correct me, but not in anger. Let no evil smite me during the day or night. Lord Jehovah come and heal all which concerns me. Remove me from the Jericho blocking my health, financial, physical or spiritual breakthrough. By the power of your holy spirit, drive away all this sickness from my body.

Banish the sickness in my body. Restore my strength and renew my body and soul. I put off all forms of fear and weakness in my life and put on the new armour, with courage and strength. I thank you for all the spiritual blessings. I tear down the stronghold of Satan and all evil that has been formed against me. I refuse to be discouraged; I claim victory. Sickness, disease, and pain I resist you in the name of Almighty God. You are not the will of God. I command you to leave my body and soul.

God make me whole; deliver and save me. Give me total victory in all my endeavours. Send new life into my body, so that goodness and mercy will follow me, today, and forevermore. Holy Spirit, anoint me with your healing power. I need you each day, and also to prepare for my tomorrow. I am free from condemnation. Your truth has set me free. You have freed me, and broken the chain of sin and oppression. Thank you for your love and your grace.

I am of the opinion that we should use our religion wisely, to go forward and progress in life, and to build us spiritually. Not as a deterrent to our general well-being or blockage of our cure, or enjoyment of life. Heaven helps those who help themselves. God provides, but you also need to put effort in the success of your own healing.

Chapter Five

Kidney Transplantation Defined

In chapter 5, part 2 of *Living a Normal and Healthy Life After Renal (Kidney) Failure,* I discuss the theoretical aspects of transplantation. A proper understanding of this chapter is essential to fully comprehend kidney transplants. This chapter defines transplants, gives reasons for kidney transplants, compares dialysis to transplants, gives types of kidney transplants, and sources of kidneys for transplants.

Kidney transplantation has dramatically improved over the years, bringing about an increase in kidney recipient survival. A remarkable improvement in the knowledge of kidney transplantation was possible due to a greater understanding of the immune system, discovery of antigens and their use, coupled with a better understanding of the kidney transplantation procedure.

If you have been diagnosed with kidney failure, to help you stay alive, you will have to be on dialysis. Kidney transplantation then becomes an option to consider. Kidney transplantation is an ongoing treatment; the recipient is required to take medication for the rest of his life. It is important to note that donated kidneys are not easy to come by, and that patients at times wait long periods to find a compatible kidney. Candidates for transplantation are patients with chronic or end stage renal failure.

Surgery is done under general anaesthesia. The kidneys are located on either side of the body, underneath the diaphragm near the lower back. The diseased kidney is not removed unless it causes discomfort.

Then the new kidney is inserted, above the top of either the right or left groin of the leg, just below the abdomen. The blood vessel from the leg is connected to the kidney for the blood flow to the kidney, and is attached to the bladder for urine passage through the urethra.

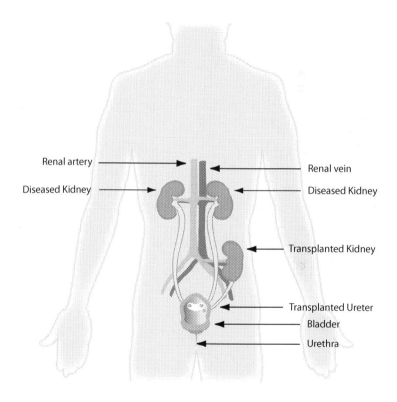

Renal artery
Diseased Kidney
Renal vein
Diseased Kidney
Transplanted Kidney
Transplanted Ureter
Bladder
Urethra

Picture of the newly transplanted kidney.

Kidneys come mainly from two sources: living donors and cadaveric. The advantages of receiving a kidney from a living donor over a cadaveric donor, are as follows:

- Waiting time for kidney recipients is being reduced, due to donated living kidneys.
- Kidneys donated by living related donors are more likely to be a good match.
- The problem associated with kidney shortage is reduced.
- Kidneys from living donors are in a better condition, as the operations are done in the same hospital, overcoming the need for transportation, and the risks involved when moving an organ from one place to the other.

LIVING RELATED — Renal transplants are donors who are related: brother, sister, parent, child, niece, nephew, aunt, uncle or cousin. Generally these transplants are more successful, as the donors are related to the recipient. (23)

LIVING UNRELATED — Renal transplants are from donors who do not share the same genetic materials as the recipient: spouse, distant relatives, friends, or an unknown donors. (24)

CADAVERIC (DECEASED) DONORS — Cadaveric donors in the United Kingdom are individuals with organ donor cards, or their families agree to donate their organs when they are confirmed dead. There are two types: heart-beating and non-heart beating.

HEART-BEATING donors are brain dead. Brain dead is defined as being unable to breathe without assistance, or on a life support machine. Once tests confirm that the brain damage is irreversible, an operation is done to remove the kidneys.

NON-HEART BEATING donors are patients that receive full resuscitation, which fails to restart the heart. Then the patient is declared dead. The patient might have suffered brain haemorrhage, a heart attack or other condition which results in cardiac arrest (heart stopping). (25)

The period of recovery after kidney transplantation is 4 to 6 weeks. The patient should avoid heavy activity during this time. The kidney recipient is usually observed for about two weeks in the hospital. After being discharged from the hospital he/she requires a close follow-up in the transplant clinic.

The survival rate for recipients of both cadaveric and live donor kidneys has dramatically improved in recent years.

Chapter Six

Positive Aspects of Kidney Transplantation

After I returned home after my transplant operation, it then properly sank into my head, the privilege of being given a new lease on life. I sobbed a lot. It was as if I was still dreaming that my life was about to change. I really thanked God, and the families of my donors, for this wonderful opportunity of a new life accorded me. Believe me; the joy in me was immeasurable. I continued to think about what this opportunity would bring into my life. My life style was about to change.

After returning home I just wanted to start a new life straight away, and get on with everything. I felt like doing everything that I had not been able to during the years that my life was brought to a standstill. I wanted to go to the cinema, and visit all my old friends at the same time; go to discos parties, and just enjoy my life again. But I was a bit cautious, as I felt things would progress naturally and needed careful planning; no need to be in a rush as I would get there eventually anyway.

Getting a kidney transplant has brought some positive changes, and results and I would like to share the positive aspects of kidney transplantation in my life.

STARTED URINATING

The first positive thing I was able to experience after my transplantation was the ability to start to urinate naturally, after 4.5 years of not being able to pass urine. It started during my weeks in the hospital, passing ¾ litre to over 2 litres a day. The feeling that my life was coming together again, and the joy that I started to feel when I wanted to urinate, after my transplant showed the success of the operation, as my kidney had started to function well.

IMPROVED KIDNEY FUNCTION

Secondly, after my transplant I had increased kidney functioning, which eventually led to me stopping dialysis. With dialysis I had a lot of horrible experiences. After treatments I was always very weak, without energy, cramps, headaches, nausea and at times feeling dizzy, coupled with psychological, emotional and stress problems. At times my mood could change drastically into depression.

INCREASED FLUID INTAKE

Now I don't have to worry about my fluid intake, meaning no fluid restrictions. Before I watched my fluid intake all the time. While I was on dialysis my allowance for daily fluid intake was half a litre. After my transplant, I started with 5 litres of fluid a day and this was lowered to 2 to 2.5 litres per day. Too much fluid pre-dialysis can eventually lead to death, as excess water in the body increases the chances of having a cardiac problem; if care is not taken this can lead to cardiac arrest. This is why your weight is monitored all the time while on dialysis.

DIET RESTRICTIONS LIFTED

With my new kidney, there are no more restrictions on my diet, though I have to be careful not to put on excessive, unwanted weight. Now I don't need to worry about the amount of water for preparing my meals, like my much loved African dishes: Amala, Eba, Poundo, yams, semolina, Jollof rice, Kenke, and kwanga.With phosphate rich foods, to prevent the level of this mineral becoming too high in my blood I have to also limit foods which are rich in potassium. But I don't have to worry about high levels of urea, as the kidney will automatically remove all of this chemical from my body.

DECREASE IN UREA AND CREATINE LEVELS

Urea and creatine have are also been reduced to acceptable level. While on dialysis, my creatine level went up to 2300 umol/L, and urea was over 175 mmol/L. Since the kidney transplant, my creatine level ranges between 127 to 185 umol/L, while my urea level ranges between 4.6 to 9 mmol/L. I also stopped the use of Alfa-Calcidol tablets for bone degeneration, and stopped having EPO injections, which helped boost my haemoglobin level. I no longer inject myself with Recopen, and stopped taking calcium deficiency tablets — Calci-Chew 500mg, Renagel Sevelamar 800 mg, and Phosex 1000mg.

CHANGES TO COMPLEXION

With my kidney transplantation another thing that was noticed in me was the changes to my skin. Everyone who saw me after my transplant noticed this improvement immediately. During my dialysis, my skin which used to be a natural black became blue-black, (I was naturally very dark), and extremely dry. This was associated with my kidney failure. There were deposits of uremic toxins that the dialysis machine could not remove. But with the transplant my skin changed back to its natural black, due to my kidney functioning normally and removing the toxic wastes in my body.

IMPROVEMENT IN SEX LIFE

After a kidney transplantation, there is an improvement in sex life. During dialysis there is a loss of sexual activity, and inability to have a proper erection. Sex life will return to normal. Chronic fatigue will diminish. The ability to get an erection will also be improved. For pre-menopausal women, the menstrual cycle will resume, and with it the possibility of becoming pregnant once again. Sexual activity becomes higher on your agenda, as you will want to make up for lost time.

NO MORE RESTRICTIONS ON DAILY ACTIVITY

Restrictions on travel are lifted. (This is severely limited while on dialysis.) People of African origin should wait for at least one year after kidney transplantation, before making the journey to Africa and need to confirm that with their transplant clinic.

With kidney failure, personal and family problems, such as stress and depression are often experienced. After the transplant you can return to work, but over a period of time, as you will need to allow the areas affected by the surgery to recover fully, and be physically fit before engaging in on full time employment.

IMPROVED PSYCHOLOGICAL HEALTH

Reconciliation is possible, conflicts with parents and children or siblings can now be reduced, and marital conflicts and problems may diminish and eventually come to be a thing of the past.

The key to positive kidney transplantation is moderation, understanding the situation, and knowing your limitations. You don't want to overdo things, though you will be tempted to try to fulfil all your worldly dreams at the same time, to make up for lost time. Be careful not to overdo things.

Chapter Seven

Problems with Kidney Transplants

Prior to my operation, I had little knowledge of kidney transplantation and what was actually involved. Having a transplant ended the transplant myth. I am not alone in this; many people, especially those from the developing countries believe that once you have your kidney transplantation, all your woes are over, everything returns to normal and you can even stop taking medication.

A friend visited me, and saw I was still taking medication. To her this was not normal, and even surprising to her. I took the time to explain to her what awaits me if I have a nonchalant attitude towards my medication, the consequences, like rejection and other things to follow. She was amazed. It seems a lot of people are ignorant about the transplantation process.

This made me want to get the message about kidney transplantation across, so that people know that after getting a new kidney, the recipient has to be very careful not to have a rejection, due to not taking enough care. I want to highlight the problems of kidney patients. The problems associated are many, but one should just keep his/her fingers crossed that they will sail through without problems.

I thought that the year 2005 was to be a year of joy for me, and that I would receive my kidney transplant, but when this did not happen, I decided to learn more about the process. Unfortunately while I was learning about the problems one might face after transplantation, the first thing I read was that of the possibility of developing cancer. This made me panic, as I did not have the slightest idea one could develop cancer after the operation. So I decided to read more. The information sent shock waves around my body, and I immediately disliked the idea of having a new kidney placed in my body. Once I was finally advised I had a donor, I was stressed and weary, but finally made up my mind to go for the operation.

What I discovered helped me to be aware of what to expect. Now I want to help others to be aware beforehand, knowing that they should be prepared for some difficulties and challenges ahead, which they will have to face and deal with. This information is not meant to discourage, or deter other renal patients from taking this wonderful opportunity, but to prepare them mentally, and to help them to be strong for the challenges they will need to cope with. I will categorise the problems into two parts. The first are those faced before and during the transplantation surgery, and the second are problems faced after the surgery.

WAITING SEVERAL YEARS FOR A MATCH

Firstly, patients waiting for a transplant operation have to be aware that there is the possibility of waiting several years before a donor match or a compatible kidney is found, unless there is a family member, friend or somebody ready to donate immediately. Everybody on the waiting list should have access to the donor kidneys, but donated kidneys in the UK are not on 'first come first served' basis, but on finding the best possible tissue match and compatibility. For people of African, Afro-Caribbean and Asian origin the waiting time is longer, due to the shortage of compatible donated kidneys.

SURGICAL PROCEDURE PROBLEMS

Secondly, there might be problems during surgery. The operation might have complications, and a lot of things could go wrong. Anybody facing this difficult time and challenge, must be prepared mentally beforehand for possible complications occurring. For example, during my own process, I was operated upon four times altogether, because I had a biopsy that went wrong, and damage to internal veins caused me to have internal bleeding. I would say that I am lucky to be alive.

UROLOGICAL COMPLICATIONS

This might arise as a result of problems during the operation, which might lead to death. Very careful attention has to be given, and precautions have to be taken, at each stage of the surgery. Kinking of the ureters are the major causes of obstruction, and a calculi stone from the donor kidney is another cause of urological complication.

URINE LEAKS

This can sometimes occur after the operation. Urine leaks are responsible for a diminished renal function which causes pain, fever and swelling. Urine leaks can also develop into intra-peritoneal leaks.

RISING CREATINE LEVEL

This may also be noticed in newly transplanted patients, due to oedema in anastomosis, and ischema infection-mucosal oedema.

VASCULAR AND LYMPATIC COMPLICATIONS

Primary problems include: renal artery thrombosis, renal vein thrombosis, renal artery stenosis, and renal vein stenosis.

Renal artery thrombosis occurs in the early post-operation period. The major reason for complications is attributed to technical errors during the kidney transplant operation. Renal vein thrombosis is caused by compression of the vein by fluid retention, also problems associated with surgical techniques.

Complications that might arise from urological and vascular lymphatic can be corrected if detected earlier. Radiologists use ultrasound, MRI, CT scan and nuclear medicine scanning methods to detect and evaluate the complications. Angiograph procedures can also be used to correct the problem.

ADAPTING TO INCREASE IN FLUID INTAKE

After the operation, it is recommended that you drink 5 litres of fluid per day, to help make the kidneys work, and flush and clean out the entire system. The problem with adjusting to drinking lots of fluid is that at times you feel like vomiting.

During my haemodialysis days my recommended fluid balance was half a litre a day. I managed with this for about six years, but with a lot of problems. Drinking 5 litres a day — ten times my previous intake — was an enormous problem to cope with.

DELAYS IN NEW KIDNEY FUNCTIONING

If the kidneys do not start functioning a few days after the operation, the transplant team starts to get worried, as this might be due to the kidney being rejected. Dialysis will be done to help eliminate the build up of toxic wastes and fluid in the body. High temperature, feeling sick, vomiting, headache, heavy stomach and other symptoms can follow.This complication is classified as acute tubular necrosis, which is due to prolonged ishema (cold or warm), and also due to reperfusion, (damage to tissue caused when blood supply returns to the tissue after a period of ischemia). The kidney not working can lead to inability to pass urine, as happened to me after the operation. It took nearly three weeks after the operation, before my kidney finally jump-started and I began to pass urine.

REJECTION

About 70% of kidney transplant patients might experience signs of rejection. The immune system of the patient sees the transplanted kidney as a foreign invader and as a threat, and eventually wants to destroy it. This is why each patient has to be monitored in the hospital. Once a rejection is detected it is possible for the body to be prevented from rejecting, before irreparable damage is done to the new kidney.

Unless the kidney comes from a related donor like a twin or other close relative, the body's reaction is to reject it as a foreign invader. Even when the matches are close, the patient will still need a life-time of immunosuppressive drugs, to suppress the immune system, increasing the risk of infection, high blood pressure, high cholesterol, and cancer.

Transplant rejection could be acute, chronic or hyper acute. Acute rejections cause painful kidneys and fever within the first year after the transplant. Chronic is where the kidney progressively declines, leading to renal failure. Hyper acute is where the kidneys fail immediately after transplantation, leading to the kidney being removed.

These problems are treated with increasing the dosage of the immunosuppressive medication. The mainstream drugs which are normally readjusted are cyclosporine, prednisolone and mycophelonate.

A sign of decreased function of the new kidney, due to rejection and the toxic effect of immunosuppressive tablets, is a drop in urine output. The creatine level and blood urine nitrogen (BUN) levels will continue to rise.

Sadly, if the kidneys do not recover, with anti-rejection treatment, the patient has to return to a life of dialysis. That is why it is so important to take the treatment very seriously, by taking all daily medication, especially anti-rejection tablets.

UTERIC STENT REMOVAL

A stent is a fine plastic tube, which is left in the body for about six weeks after the new kidney transplant, to help the flow of urine from the new kidney. The uteric stent is removed under local anaesthetic, with an antibiotic injection to protect against infection. After, a mild burning sensation is often noticed in patients while passing urine, which soon gets better, and blood may be noticed in the urine, which is common.

INFECTIONS

Renal patients with transplants are faced with a high risk of infection, or cancer, attributed to the immunosuppressive therapy, which is used to suppress the immune system. Pulmonary infections, urinary tract infections, wound infections, infections of the gastrointestinal tract, and reoccurrence of Hepatitis B are the most common.

PULMONARY INFECTION is related to respiration. For example, chronic bronchitis, or airway obstruction. Pulmonia in renal patients leads to morbidity, and death.

URINARY TRACT INFECTION leads to the increase of bacteraemia in renal patients.

WOUND INFECTIONS are related to surgical problems during the transplant operation.

VIRAL INFECTIONS might be transmitted by the donated kidney, self inflicted, or due to a careless sex life.

HEPATITIS B VIRUS can occur in renal patients with a history of, or currently with hepatitis infections. HBV DNA shows up after transplantation, indicating active viral replication.

CANCER

The development of cancer after transplantation in renal patients is quite unfortunate. Skin cancer is most prevalent. Transplant patients are advised to avoid excessive sun exposure, sun bathing, and not use sun tanning beds, to help prevent skin cancer and damage to the skin cells. The sun's rays are agents of skin cancer. The dermatologist often looks for signs of skin cancer, especially in patients of African descent.

SKIN CANCER is due to over-exposure to the sun, in combination with the immunosuppressant medication. The two types of cancer are Squamous Cell Cancer (SCC1) and Basal Cell Cancer (BCC1). The two types often appear as lumps, ulcers, red patches, on the face, neck, scalp, ears, and lips. The more serious form of cancer is called Malignant Melanoma.

The human herpes virus type 8 (hhv8) viruses starts skin cancer. There might be a noticed swelling, or dark spots on the legs, or dark patches or lumps might appear on the legs. If any of these occur, the renal doctor will have to reduce immunosuppressant medications, and keep monitoring.

In other to avoid skin cancer, renal and transplant patients are advised to observe the following:
- Keep away from the sun in as much as possible.
- In extreme sun, wear hat and sunglasses.
- Wear long sleeved clothes.
- Wear a strong sun screen cream to protect the body from the sun.

SKIN WARTS
The other type of dermatological problem. Warts are due to an infection of the skin, caused by a virus. Common in all areas of the body exposed to the sun.

DENTAL PROBLEMS
Another problem often faced after transplantation is mouth ulcers, which, if not treated, can lead to mouth cancer. Mouth ulcers are painful sores that appear inside the mouth.

Mine developed initially as a small dot on my tongue. After some time my gums got swollen and prevented me from eating; I had to restrict myself to soup, for several months. The ulcer spread all over my tongue and entire gums. It was like wild fire, as my tongue and gums became unbearable with pain. Then I developed a constant headache. I used plenty of the recommended mouth wash and tablets, but none seem to address the situation, so I was referred to a specialist dentist.

On the day of my mouth biopsy, the tongue was numbed with a local anaesthetic. My mouth was operated on to remove the ulcerated layers on my tongue, afterwards, the tongue was stitched back together. The sutures would dissolve after about ten days, the surgeon told me. After the operation, I was advised to avoid brushing the tongue, as this may cause irritation in the area operated upon, and delay healing. The layers removed were later sent to the laboratory to check for mouth cancer. The results confirmed that it was not mouth cancer, but an inflammation. I was greatly relieved upon hearing this.

MOUTH CANCER can appear in any part of the mouth, on tongue, gums, lips, or in the throat. People can also die from mouth cancer. That is why the earlier the detection, the earlier the treatment, the better. Smoking tobacco cigarettes or chewing paan with tobacco, are major causes of mouth cancers. Transplant patients need to visit a dentist regularly, to check for signs of mouth cancer.

CONSTANT NIGHT SWEATING

Another problem I noticed after my transplant was constant sweating at night, in bed. I never used to sweat at all while sleeping. But since I had my transplant I continuously sweat while sleeping making the bed wet.

EXCESSIVE HAIR GROWTH

I also noticed excessive hair growth all over my body. This is unusual for me. This was due to the steroids I was taking. I now shave every day.

CHANGES TO PHYSICAL APPEARANCE

You might develop a 'round face' over time, and other changes to your physical appearance, due to the immunosuppressants used to treat the problem of rejection.

EAR, NOSE AND THROAT (ENT) PROBLEMS

I also developed ear, nose and eye problems. My nose was constantly blocked, with my eye balls watery, swollen and red all the time. My hearing was also impaired. I still cannot figure out whether the constant nose blockage was due to my kidney transplant or not. I was referred to the ENT clinic, where an operation was booked. On the day of the operation, I developed high blood pressure, which meant the operation was delayed, as my blood pressure needed to be normalised first.

As there was no big improvement in the high blood pressure, it was decided by the surgical team that I be operated on under a local anaesthesthetic, rather than a general anaesthetic to avoid the complications that might arise with general anaesthesia. The operation was successfully done with a Grommet (small object to aid hearing and discharge of unwanted fluid) in my ear. Thanks to the medical team, and glory be to God. For my constant blocked nose, I used Fluticasone Aqu nasal spray 50 mcg, two squirts into both nostrils each day, to help ease the problem.

ADJUSTING AFTER TRANSPLANTATION

The problems associated with adjusting to a new life after receiving a new kidney, are also worth mentioning. After being given a new lease of life, the transplant recipient needs to make adjustments; to live with the new kidney. There is also the emotional issue, knowing that if the donated kidney starts to lose functioning, that the kidney will eventually fail.

Chapter Eight

Diet for Kidney Transplant Patients

In part 1, chapter 9, of *Living a Normal and Healthy Life After Renal (Kidney) Failure,* I discuss at length, diet for kidney failure patients. This chapter is a continuation — for newly transplanted patients. After kidney transplantation, diet has a significant role to play; to assist full recovery from the operation, and to regain strength. This means prioritising dietary needs. But eating should now be a thing of pleasure, not discomfort.

After you have recovered fully from your kidney operation, there is the possibility of an increase in your eating, as you will want to eat as much as you like, now that your appetite has improved again. The previous limitations, due to kidney failure, on what you can eat will usually be relaxed quite quickly. But you have to get your diet right, so that you keep yourself and your new kidney as healthy as possible.

I will share my experience with this issue. The first week after I left the hospital was the birthday of my son, Kenneth. I was waiting anxiously for this day. The family decided to go to a Chinese café for the occasion, an eat-as-much-as-you-like buffet. The atmosphere of the restaurant was brilliant and there was so much to eat. Being the first time eating properly after my transplant, I was fascinated by the amount of food suddenly available for me to eat. So I started with soup and after went for the main course, ending with ice cream. Before I realised what was happening, I had already overeaten, to the extent that I found it difficult to even stand up.

We left the restaurant and went home. On getting to the house, I was very uncomfortable. I was praying that the food would quickly digest in my stomach, but things were not moving as well as I hoped. When the time to sleep approached, I was very agitated, and could not sleep till the following morning. To tell the truth, I had only myself to blame, because when I saw the selection in the restaurant I wanted to have a bit of everything. This was due to the food restrictions during my early days of dialysis, which I now wanted to compensate for. Since that day, I promised myself I would take it a little easier with food.

Because of the temptations, after the food restrictions are lifted, you have to be very careful, and keep an eye on yourself, otherwise you will want to over-eat, to make up for lost time. Diet, in renal transplant patients, is all about healthy eating. Healthy eating is about a gradual change in your eating behaviour. With healthy food choices, you can eat almost everything — in moderation. Healthy foods are low in fat and sugar, and high in complex carbohydrate: cereals, vegetables and grains, fresh fruits and vegetables, fish and other proteins. You should abstain from fatty foods.

Note that a healthy diet:

-Prevents excessive weight gain.
-Prevents the build up of cholesterol, so it is within normal limits, which helps keep the heart healthy.
-Helps keep sugar level within desirable limits, which ultimately can prevent diabetes.
-Helps keep blood pressure normal.
-Helps make the bones stronger, with the required amount of calcium.

If you are in the habit of eating excessively, this can make you gain a lot of weight. Weight gain in transplant patients is common. You might gain up to 10 kilos within a short period of time, after transplantation, if care is not taken. Gaining weight is easier than losing it. It is advisable to weigh yourself every other day, to monitor changes in your weight. If you notice a weight gain start immediately with diet changes, begin doing light exercise, and if possible see your dietician immediately, for consultation on your diet.

In other to avoid gaining too much weight:

- Reduce portions of foods eaten.
- Eat more vegetables, as they are low in calories.
- Try to be more active. Go for a walk or cycle; being active will keep you happy and healthy.

Apart from excessive eating, medications like Cyclosporine and Prednisolone reduce the body's ability to convert sugar to energy, which means that the sugar level in your body will rise, which can lead to steroid induced diabetes. These also increase appetite and lead to fluid retention. The combination of weight gain and steroids gives rise to high blood pressure, and increase in coronary heart disease, due to high cholesterol or high triglycerides, hypertension, obesity, blood vessel disease, and risk of developing diabetes, so it is advisable to reduce fat in the diet. Try to avoid concentrated sugar. Being overweight puts a lot of strain on your body, which eventually can contribute to health problems.

Eating healthy includes proper food storage. When you buy chilled or frozen foods take them home quickly and store them in the fridge/freezer at the correct temperature, follow the manufacturer's instructions, as indicated inside the fridge and freezer.

Wash your hands properly when you go to the toilet, handle rubbish, or touch pets before handling your foods. Cook food properly. Store cooked food and raw food separately. Do not store cooked food for more than a few days, as mould begins to develop. Guard against food poisoning by checking the 'use by' dates, and always use within the recommended time frame.

GUIDELINES FOR HEALTHY EATING

- Eat high fibre foods: fruit, vegetables, whole grains, beans and lentils.
- Eat food high in calcium; milk, cheese, yoghurt, salmon, sardines, green leafy vegetables.
- Avoid foods high in sugar: fruit juices, soda, fizzy drinks, chocolates, sweets, and ice cream.
- Use artificial sweeteners instead of sugar.
- Avoid salt if possible. Do not add salt at the table. Salts increase the body's ability to retain fluids, raising blood pressure. Avoid: commercial soups, salted, bottled pickles, olives, onions, soy sauce and processed meat; salted fish, like panla, makayabu or okporoko.
- Avoid foods high in listeria: unpasteurized cheese, pate, live yogurt and food containing raw eggs, e.g. mayonnaise. Listeria bacteria can cause problems when taking higher doses of anti-rejection drugs.
- Avoid frying foods; try to grill, bake or steam.
- Choose lean meat, and remove all visible fat before cooking.
- Avoid foods rich in fat: fried foods, sausage, full fat dairy products, chicken skin, bacon, and junk food, such as pizza or crisps.
- Limit butter, margarine, red meat.
- Choose poly-saturated rather than saturated fat.
- Limit egg yolks to three times per week. Cook eggs thoroughly, and avoid foods containing raw eggs.

- Eat more fish, including a portion of oily fish each week. Fish is an excellent source of protein and contain many vitamins and minerals. Oily fish contains Omega 3 fatty acids, which can help keep the heart healthy.

- Eat more fruit and vegetables, at least 5 portions of either every day.

- Eat high protein foods. Protein is important for building and repairing muscles and tissues, which helps prevent muscle weakness due to high doses of Prednisolone; it also assists healing after surgery.

- Avoid soft ripened cheese like Brie, Camembert, Stilton and Mascarpone.

- Keep intake of alcohol within safe limits.

Enjoy what you eat, whilst having a varied diet. Strive to maintain a healthy weight for your size.

Nutritional requirements will vary for different races, after a kidney transplant. Nutritional guidelines should be tailored to each person's specific requirements. Please note that the information given is general guidance on diet and transplantation. You will need to work with your dietician to work out the best dietary plan for your needs; after a transplant, several dietary changes are necessary.

Chapter Nine

Medication for Kidney Transplant Patients

The issue of medication in newly transplanted patients is very critical. That is why I have chosen to highlight and shed more light on this. To give the new kidney a chance to survive and to keep you healthy, you will need to understand that you cannot be lazy with taking your medication, or have a nonchalant attitude.

I want to use this chapter to correct the misconception that when you have a kidney transplant everything is fine, everything returns to normal; there is no longer any need to continue to take any medication, as at last you are free from daily medication.

This is not true. Now that you have a new kidney you have to take your medication very seriously. A 'don't care' attitude will kill the new kidney. I will give you an instance. A friend, very religious, visited me after my kidney transplant. She saw me still taking a lot of tablets after I returned home from the hospital. This was very surprising to her. She took courage and said, "But your kidney is now working isn't it?" I answered, "Yes." The next thing she told me was, "The Lord has answered your prayer; you don't need to take all this medication any more."

I tried to explain to her the importance of taking my medication and the risks which I would face by not doing the right thing. To this she said, "The Lord has taken action and control. Soon you will not need to take all this medication any longer. In the name of the Lord." As she refused to understand my explanation and point of view, I left her with her opinion, as I was just recovering from my operation and don't want to be involved in a long discussion on the matter. As I said earlier, a lot of people confuse the realities of life with their religious beliefs.

The importance of your medication should not be underestimated. Remember that these drugs serve a very important function in the body. For newly transplanted kidney patients, the issue of medication cannot be taken lightly. This is the time you have to exercise self discipline, determination and willpower. You cannot be lazy, complacent or forgetful with taking your medication at the right time and the recommended dose. You cannot develop a habit of skipping your medication either.

Remember, you waited a long time for this glorious opportunity of your life — to have a kidney transplant. If you are of an ethnic minority group, you probably waited twice or three times longer for a compatible kidney, due to the shortage of donor kidneys. So this is not the time to make mistakes. If you do not take your medication on time and as prescribed, this can have fatal consequences.

As there are a lot of pills to take each day, at times you will be fed up, tired and not want to bother, but you have to understand that you don't want to be inconsistent with your medication. Because of your condition, you need to take different types of pills, and you should not minimise the value of any of them.

I suggest you buy pill reminders, sold at any chemist: daily, weekly and monthly reminders, with three or four compartments, for breakfast, lunch, dinner and bedtime.

Immunosuppressive tablets are used to prevent rejection which arises as a result of inflammation (swelling) of the kidney. These are very powerful drugs, used to make the immune system less effective, so that the transplanted kidney is not rejected. Given in large doses immediately after kidney transplant, reduced and readjusted when the kidney has started working properly. These are taken for as long as the kidney is functioning.

The immunosuppressive tablets have to be taken at the right time and at the prescribed dosage. Your kidney might be rejected if you don't take these, causing you to have to return to a life of dialysis. That is why I continue to stress that you need to take your medication seriously.

Medications to suppress the immune system have some long-term side effects, which include: high blood pressure, glucose intolerance, diabetes, and weight gain, increased risk of infection, tumours, osteoporosis, muscle weakness and cataract formation in the eyes.

There are various medications available for the prevention of rejection, and keeping you healthy. Most transplant clinics use a combination of immunosuppressants to prevent rejection. These are adjusted after blood check results at the transplant clinic, so as to have the right amount of the medication in the blood stream.

Note: High levels of immunosuppressants lead to toxicity, while low levels can cause rejection.

The following drugs were prescribed for me, after discharge from hospital, after a successful kidney transplant: (26)

- Cyclosporine (Neural 200 mg bd)
- MMF (Cellcept) Mycophenolate Mofetil 1.5 bd
- Prednisolone 20 mg od
- Co-trimoxazole 480 mg bd

- Valganciclovil 480 mg twice weekly
- Amlodipin 10 mg nocte later changd to Doxazon tablets 4 mg, 2 tablets twice daily
- Atorvasatin 20 mg nocte
- Erythropoietin (neorecormon) Pen 5000, twice per week.
- Pregabalin 25 mg nocte
- Tramadol 50 tds prn
- Ranitidine 150 mg nocte
- Calcichew D 3 Forte 2 tablets od
- Folic acid 5 mg od
- Aspirin 75 mg od
- Paracetamol 1 g qds pm
- Lactulose 20 mls bd pm
- Senna 2 tablets bd prn

Most medicines prescribed after kidney transplant have led to good results. You will have to follow the medication plan as recommended. The doctor will continue to monitor you and your blood results and make necessary adjustments to your dosage.

Here are more details on each type of medication.

CYCLOSPORIN – An immunosuppressive, which prevents the body from producing certain types of cells that contribute to kidney rejection. Dosage depends on the level of cyclosporine in the blood.

Side effects: increased blood pressure; excessive hair growth; overgrowth of gum tissues; increased level of the cholesterol in the body; damage to liver and kidney; feeling tired; tingling.

MYCOPHELONAT – Immunosuppressive. Note, your body will be prone to life-threatening infection, if too much is taken. Side effects: constipation; urinary tract infection; abdominal pain; diarrhoea; vomiting; upper respiratory infection.

PREDNISONE – Immunosuppressive which helps to reduce inflammation, which is part of rejection. Side effects: changes in the appearance, such as round face; diabetes; joint problems; stomach ulcers; weight gain; cataracts; hypertension; acne.

The aforementioned immunosuppressant drugs have the side effects of one being prone to infection, or developing skin cancer, flu, or pneumonia. If you notice chills or fever, you should report this to your transplant clinic. To be on the safe side, do not skip a dose, or change your medication without consulting your doctor.

Also, consult your doctor if you want to take any over-the-counter medication, as these may interfere with your drugs. Report any side effects to your doctor.

CO-TRIMOXAZOLE – Prescribed for the first three months after kidney transplantation. Recommended to help avoid developing certain types of chest infection, urinary tract infection, ear infection, bacterial infection that cause abscesses, and toxoplasmosis, which comes from eating undercooked meat. Side Effects: skin rash; swelling of the face, lips, tongues; difficulty breathing; fast heartbeat; inflamed heart or blood vessels; muscle or joint pain.

VULGANCICLORIL – Used to help prevent viral infection and to heal a serious eye infection. Also recommended to be used usually for 3 months, after the kidney transplant operation. Side effects: nausea, diarrhoea and abdominal pain.

AMLODIPIN – Used in treatment of high blood pressure, to relax the blood vessels so that the blood passes through them easily. Also for reducing the possibility of angina, whilst suffering from chest pain. Side effects: headache; peeling and blistering of the skin and mouth; dizziness and fatigue; flushing; ankles swelling; rash affecting the whole body. Your blood pressure tablets may be increased if you develop high blood pressure after your kidney transplant.

When I went for the dressing on my fistula,I started to feel uncomfortable, so I told the nurse to help measure my blood pressure. I was lucky she did. My blood pressure had soared to 230/125. So I was immediately sent to the transplant clinic for further investigation. Blood pressure lowering drugs were immediately prescribed: Rampiril, 10mg; Atenol, 50mg; Doxazon, 8 mg twice daily. The blood pressure then improved, to a reasonable level.

ATOVASTATIN – Also known as Lipitor – drug used to help lower cholesterol build up in the body, help prevent cardiovascular disease, blocks the enzymes that control the rate of cholesterol production in the body, can increase the good cholesterol and decrease bad cholesterol, and helps to reduce fatty substances in the body called triglyceride lipid fats.

ERYTHROPOIETIN – This injection is used to boost the bone marrow to retain sufficient red blood cells levels, and boost haemoglobin level, also used to treat anaemia. Once the kidney starts to function properly, this will no longer be needed, as the new kidney automatically produces this substance for the body.

PREGABALIN – An anticonvulsant drug used to treat neuropathic pain, chronic pain, also to treat general anxiety. Side Effects: memory impairment; erectile dysfunction; depression; confusion; agitation; hallucination; dizziness; drowsiness; blurred vision.

TRAMADOL – Pain reliever which helps treats moderate, severe and chronic pain. Overconsumption of this drug can lead to convulsions, sleeping problems, blurred vision, nausea and vomiting, weak pulse and rashes.

RANITIDIN – also called Histamine 2 Blockers. Helps reduce skin irritation, and constant heart burn, and helps to also prevent indigestion. Also used to treat ulcers in the stomach and intestine, and gastric ulcers. Side effects: headache; dizziness; diarrhoea; and rash.

CALCI-CHEW D3 FORTE – Contains two active ingredients. Calcium carbonate supplements calcium in the diet. Vitamin D3 is used for the formation of strong bones and healthy teeth, also to transmit nerve signals in the body; too much of it in the body is called hypocalcaemia. Discontinued shortly after kidney transplantation.

FOLIC ACID – A special vitamin supplement which helps in the formation of red and white blood cells and helps to treat anaemia.

ASPIRIN – Helps thin the blood and prevent clots forming in blood vessels, prevents heart attack and strokes, anti-inflammatory, helps in treating aches and pain. Side effects: stomach irritation, and indigestion.

PARACETAMOL – Pain reliever, also helps in reducing fever. Serious side effects if taken in large doses.

LACTULOSE – Synthetic sugar used to treat constipation, helps to empty the stomach, helps treat a complicated liver disease. Side effects: abdominal cramping; gas; diarrhoea.

SENNA – Used in treating constipation, as a stimulating laxative. Side effects: stomach cramps, and pain.

NOTE:
Non-prescribed drugs should not be used without consulting your transplant clinic doctor, as some non-prescribed medication can be dangerous, or interfere with your medication.

Chapter Ten

Organ Donations for Kidney Transplant Patients

Organ donor shortage is a universal problem. The problem has brought to light the difficulties encountered while waiting for kidneys for patients with chronic or end-stage renal failure. Also accompanying problems, like a shortage of transplant specialists, as many opt out of finishing their internship, due to the extremely heavy workload.

In part 1, pages 84 – 85, I talked about this problem, and various barriers to organ donor shortage in ethnic minority groups, especially African, Afro-Caribbean and Asian.

The main issue is how we encourage more people from the black and Asian communities to join the Organ Transplant Register to donate. There should be a campaign to encourage people to sign up for donor cards.

I encourage everyone to get a donor card, by registering at the NHS Organ Register: telephone 08456 0604000 for details, or register on line at www.uktransplant.org.uk

******

I would like to share my experience whilst in the transplant ward, waiting for a kidney transplant.

Within the white community, there appears to be a greater tendency to donate for their friends or family; giving the gift of a lifetime. Seeing the suffering, pain and agony of loved one on dialysis treatment, and the desire to save them their lives has made a lot of them come forward to donate. They know that they can live with one kidney, so they are willing to help their loved one survive. During my stay, I noticed at least eight white people coming to donate for their loved ones, whilst I never saw a single black or Asian person donate for a loved one.

I kept on asking myself why? It was at this juncture that I saw the disproportion. It was glaringly obvious clear that people from African, Afro-Caribbean and Asian communities either are scared or are not properly informed of the process.

Most of us from the ethnic minority depend on cadaveric donors. That is why those of ethnic minority wait longer for a transplant, on average four years or more before they find a match. I kept on wondering where our sympathy, empathy and caring disappeared to? If you are sick with kidney failure, you need a donor to help you out, and if you don't receive a kidney in time, you eventually die. But mothers, fathers, brothers, sisters, husbands, wives, etc. are too scared to donate for their loved ones.

Many tell you to just keep on praying, one day the Lord will listen to you and reward you with a kidney. This is a real religious belief. But, the question that comes to my mind with this attitude is, how will you be blessed if you are *not* offered a kidney and helped out of the horrible situation you find yourself in? You depend on a cadaveric donor, or eventually die while waiting.

The Lord will jump start the kidney, but don't wait for a miracle; too many wait endlessly, and eventually die in the process.

We, the African community, need to educate our people on the importance and positives of donating. I have seen situations where mothers prevent their children from donating for each other. As an example of this situation, there were two brothers, and one had kidney failure and needed a kidney to keep him alive. The other brother was ready to donate for his sibling, but the mother would not allow it. She was afraid that if something happened to both of them, she would be left to care for the grandchildren alone. I could understand her fears and concerns, due to her not being properly informed about the process of transplantation. The second brother eventually summoned up the courage — without informing his mother — and donated to his brother, despite their mother's objection. Thanks to improvements in the transplantation procedure, and God, the operation went well and both are now both still living and well.

We need to re-educate our people, spread the word that it is possible to live a normal life with one kidney. We need to increase the numbers of kidneys available for transplants. This could be achieved by introducing the following:

Presumed Consent/Opt out System

This works on the presumption that someone is willing to donate, unless they declare their intention not to, by specifying their objection. Prospective donors are informed of their right to opt out at any stage. This could help resolve the problem of organ shortages and the long waiting list.

Spain is a good example of a success with the opt out system. Other European countries that practise the opt out system are: Austria; Belgium; Sweden; Denmark; Finland;

France; Italy; Norway; and in Asia, Singapore. Each operate the opt out system based on their own systems and laws.

In Spain, the system has made public the aspect of human generosity in the midst of grief, whereby the views of the family are sought, as they consider whether to donate or not. Spain has a national network of specially trained doctors who speak to the bereaved families, and the waiting transplant patient. (27) Donations in Spain doubled, to 35 people per 1 million, since the introduction of the system. (28)

Spanish singer Tito Nora had a kidney transplant some years ago. She recorded a song, *Vivo por Ti,* to persuade more families to consent to organ donation. We could use our celebrities to help spread the message of becoming an organ donor. (29)

Palomar Gonzalez Lopez was a 45-year-old Spanish woman, whose father, immediately after her death, gave consent to donate her kidney. When asked why he agreed to this, he answered, "To be able to give someone the chance of life is real satisfaction. It makes you feel proud. This is everything in life. Anyone who can donate should do it, so that in the long run you'll feel happy and contented." (30)

Austria operates a 'strict' opt out system, and here the views of the relative are not taken into account. The country passed the Presumed Consent Law in 1992. Donations quadrupled, and since then the number of kidney donations each year nearly equalled the number of people on the waiting list. (31)

Sweden also operates an opt out system, but it has failed to have a significant effect on donation. The donation rate has been lower than that of the United Kingdom, suggesting other issues may have an effect on the opt out system. (32)

The following could help increase the number of kidneys for transplants:

1. Increase the number of transplant coordinators, to help transplant teams deal with workload. (33)

2. Set up a system of 'conditional' organ donation, where the donor sets up his /her conditions before death, that will be applied to the organ donated. It should be stressed that conditions for organ donation should not be set on racist or discriminatory grounds. (34)

3. A financial reward scheme to boost organ donation should also be considered. By giving financial incentive, there is an expectation that many donors might join the organ register. However there are downsides to this:

- It will put poor people in a vulnerable condition, which might lead to exploitation.
- It will increase the problem of human organ trafficking.
- Wealthy people will buy their own organs.
- Relatives of prospective donors might abuse the system by shortening the time a patient is on life support.

It is quite unfortunate; many people from developing countries have been conned to part with their organs, and later paid a petty amount of money for this. The weak are already being exploited with this system. This is termed commercial selling of organs, which is prohibited in the United Kingdom. (35)

Chapter Eleven

A Normal, Healthy Life after Organ Transplant

This chapter concludes parts 1 and part 2, of *Living a Normal and Healthy Life after Renal (Kidney) Failure.*

As I said in earlier chapters, a lot of people believe that after kidney transplantation, the mystery surrounding their health problems are over. But I tell you from experience that is not the situation. I am dispelling the myth that after transplantation you are free from any other problem related to kidney functioning.

Without a well thought out after care plan after your transplantation, you risk losing the kidney. This new kidney is an opportunity of a life time, an opportunity to be able to live a normal life. The most frightening after kidney transplantation is the possibility of rejection, which might occur if you are not taking proper care of your kidney, due to a nonchalant attitude or carelessness.

Remember how long you were on the waiting list before you finally had the chance to have a kidney transplant? I could never contemplate going back to a life of dialysis. Although some people prefer dialysis to kidney transplants. I don't, which is why I decided to highlight the issue of after care.

After kidney transplantation, if the kidneys do not start working immediately, you will need to be dialysed to help cleanse the body, especially the blood. After my kidney transplant, it took nearly three weeks before my new kidney eventually started functioning. I was continuously dialysed during that time, to remove the accumulated toxic waste in my body.

Post-transplant care entails the transplant clinic providing ongoing monitoring, and necessary information to guide patients, to enable them to live a healthy life and maintain a functioning kidney.

You will have to visit the transplant clinic regularly, starting with twice a week, then it start to diminish to once a week, once a fortnight, monthly, three-monthly, then every six months, etc. When you visit the clinic, you can expect the following:

- Blood test.
- Physical examination.
- X rays, as needed.
- Review of medications.
- Dermatological examination. (Any necessary treatment done by a dermatologist, after referral.)
- Dental examination, as needed.
- Ear, nose and throat examination, as needed.
- Eye examination, as needed.

When you are discharged from the hospital after the kidney transplant operation, you should commit to doing everything necessary to look after your kidney, so as to return to a normal life. This will include things like having an easily accessible medical identification record, with your name, telephone number of transplant clinic and your GP, and all medications, especially immunosuppressant drugs, and dosage.

Kidney transplantation after care is about total transformation of your life, from a life of dialysis to a totally different life, and being able to do a lot of things which you were not able to do while on dialysis.

To be able to maintain a healthy and working kidney, after care plays a vital role. An effective programme will help in maintaining the stability of your new kidney, and your general wellbeing. The problem which you might face by not maintaining proper after care is kidney rejection.

After care looks at various aspects of maintaining a good quality of life:

- Medication and clinical tests
- Diet. Do not make a habit of overeating as this will bring unwanted weight gain.
- Avoiding smoking and sun bathing.
- Do everything in moderation.
- Embark on regular exercise, like jogging, walking, swimming, etc.

One of the benefits of after care is being able to spot early symptoms, if rejection is about to occur. The transplant team can then take positive steps to stop the rejection.

In the initial stages after transplant, ultra sound tests are normally performed, to ensure that the main blood vessels leading to the kidney are functioning well, and that enough blood is supplied to the kidney for effective functioning. Also the ultrasound will detect any obstructions preventing blood flow to the kidney, or the accumulation of fluid around the kidney.

BLOOD TEST RESULTS SAMPLE

TABLE 1

Date	Hb	WBC	Hct	Plt	Na	K	cCa	P	AP	Tbili	Ur	Cr	CyA	Alb	Glu	C
22/07/09	12.8	5.7	0.4	180	138	3.9	2.6	0.79	79	15	8.3	145	173	48	6.2	3.9
23/05/09	12.8	4.3	0.4	175	145	4.4	2.39	0.71	92	15	9	146	471	48	5.8	3.6
19/05/09	12.8	4.5	0.4	184	146	4.1	2.55	0.76	85	15	9.5	159	156	49	7.1	3.5
28/04/09	12.2	3.2	0.35	177	145	3.8	2.65	0.73	72	11	6.5	131	186	45	5.6	3.2
24/03/09	11.6	5.4	0.35	182	145	4	2.52	0.87	79	9	7.5	142	137	45	5.6	3.7
24/02/09	10	9.9	29	212	144	4	2.51	0.85	69	7	6.8	129	140	43	5.4	2.9
27/01/09	10.5	3.2	0,31	212	144	4.2	2.59	0.64	66	8	4.6	151	113	44	7.9	2.9
30/12/08	10.5	5.4	0.32	216	144	4.7	2.58	0.84	80	7	7.3	160	118	43	5	3

Transplant Clinic Selected Cumulative Blood Results (Dec 2008–July 2009).

NOTE: The full meaning of the following parameters
Hb; WBC; Hct; Plt; Na; K; cCa; P; AP; Tbili: Ur; Cr; CyA; Alb; Glu; and C are seen in Table 2.

Your blood will be drawn during your clinic visit and sent to the laboratory for analysis the same day. Remember not to take your immunosuppressant tablets twelve hours before the blood is taken for analysis, as this might affect the results. The laboratory tests will monitor your kidney function, blood count, electrolytes and level of medication in your blood.

Below is a typical blood test result of a transplant patient. Here you will see that the blood results are not the same each time the blood was drawn. In order to maintain a normal functioning kidney, the transplant clinic keeps an eye on both blood and urine results.

SELECTED BLOOD TEST ELEMENTS AND RANGES FOR THE NEW KIDNEY		
TABLE 2		
NO	EVENT	RANGE
1	Haemoglobin (Hb) g/dL	13.5 – 17.5
2	White blood counts (WBC)/L	4 – 11
3	Haematocrit (Hct)/L	0.4 – 0.54
4	Platelet count (Plt)/L	150 – 400
5	Sodium serum (Na) mmol/L	136 – 146
6	Potassium serum (K) mmol/L	3.5 – 5.1
7	Calcium serum (cCa) mmol/L	2.15 – 2.65
8	Phosphate serum (Po) mmol/L	0.8 – 1.5
9	Alkaline Phosphate serum (AP) IU/L	40 – 129
10	Total Bilirubin serum (Tbili) umol/L	1 – 17
11	Urea (Ur) mmol/L	3.7 – 6.4
12	Creatinine (Cr) umol/L	62 – 106
13	Cyclosporine blood (CyA) microgram/L	90 – 150
14	Albumin serum (Alb) g/L	35 – 50
15	Glucose (Glu) mmol/L	2.8 – 11
16	Cholesterol C mmol/L	0 – 5

According to table 1, the **haemoglobin** level improved from 10.5 g/dl from December, 2008 and kept on improving to 12.8 g/dl in July, 2009.

The **creatine** and **urea** levels show how the kidney is functioning. A drastic rise in creatine level indicates problems with the kidney and a possibility of rejection. In men, higher levels of creatine level are often noticed, because they generally have more skeletal muscle mass than women. Another thing taken into consideration while looking at the level of creatine is race. In the black ethnic minority group, high levels of creatine are common. Also, vegetarians have been shown to have lower creatine levels. Some drugs, like ACE inhibitors, or Angiotensin, used to treat erectile dysfunction, can cause creatine levels to rise. The recommended creatine level ranges between 62 – 106 umol/L. The minimum is 129/umol/L and the maximum is 159 umol/L. These test results are still within the recommended range, as the person is black, of African origin, and male.

The **urea** is a small molecule produced in the liver from dietary protein, and becomes part of the waste products removed from the blood by the kidneys. A rise in blood levels of urea indicates a fall in kidney function. Other things that can change the level of urea in your blood are: amount of protein consumed; liver disease, and consuming too little fluid, causing your kidneys to keep more urea in your blood. Table 1 shows the Min urea level to be 4.6 mmol/L, while the Max within the test period is 9.5 mmol/L.

White blood cells (WBC), HCT, PLTS, are the parameters used for measuring the blood count. An increase in the WBC shows there is an infection; a decrease is an indication of lower defence against infection. The WBC increasing to 9.9/L in February, 2009, might not be a sign of rejection but a result of the effects of the steroids and other medication.

The **HCT** measures the amount of red blood cells in the blood. The red blood cells carry oxygen to all parts of the body. With a low HCT you feel tired, with less energy. In February, 2009 it was 0.29/L Min HCT while the other months have a range of 0.31/L – 0.41/L as the Max.

The **PLTS** measures the level of platelets in the blood. Platelets are cells that make your body form blood clots when you are injured. If the numbers are low, the possibility of serious bleeding increases. The Min of 177/L is noticed while the Max is 216/L which is still within the recommended range of 150/L – 400/L.

Sodium (Na) is the amount of salt in the body. Too much sodium in the blood causes high blood pressure, heart failure and pulmonary oedema. A lot of sodium makes you thirsty, and it is advisable to continue to drink water until the level becomes normal. The level of sodium in December, 2008 was 144 mmol/L and increased to 146 mmol/L and fell to 138 mmol/L in July, 2009. The range should be between 136 – 146 mmol/L, which is okay for the period studied.

Calcium, phosphorus, magnesium, potassium and sodium are electrolytes, which are natural minerals that get dissolved in our blood. These are also closely monitored by the transplant clinic and if adjustments are necessary, supplemented. All the indexes here are within the recommended ranges.

The **alkaline phosphate** serum and the total **Bilirubin** serum are also within the targeted ranges.

The **Cyclosporine** blood was noticed to be extremely high in June, 2009, up to 471 microgram/L, due to the fact that the patient took a steroid tablet the morning before the blood test, causing a significant increase. Otherwise the level is within the necessary range.

Albumin (Alb) g/L. This is a blood protein. Some things that can cause low levels are urine leakage, liver disease, inflammation of the kidney, poor diet, and starvation. The Min here is 43 g/L and the Max is 49 g/L, also within the ranges recommended.

Glucose (sugar) is also monitored to be sure that it is at the right level. The glucose level increasing to 7.9 mmol/L could be as a result of consuming sugary drinks, and eating a lot of refined carbohydrates, too many cakes, etc.

The **cholesterol** level is within the recommended range, and the best result was in January, 2009 where it went down to 2.8 mmol/L while the Max is 3.9mmol/L. The recommended level should not be more than 5 mmol/L.

Overall the blood results do not show too much deviation from the expected result, taking the circumstances of the patient into account, meaning the result is within expected limits and improvements are possible.

At the transplant clinic the staff will look at a combination of the above results and parameters, to analyse and determine the effectiveness and functionality of the newly transplanted kidney, and how to adjust the medications recommended.

As a newly transplanted patient, if you develop any symptoms, like fever, chills, cough, sore throat, or cloudy urine, you should report straight to the transplant clinic for examination, as this might be a sign of infection. This is quite common; as you take steroids to lower your immune system, this makes you more prone to infection.

To be more active, make regular exercise part of your day-to-day activities. The exercise can include, jogging, walking long distance, or riding a stationary bicycle — which I am now using. You should abstain from strenuous exercise, like weight lifting.

Take it easy with yourself. Allow your body to settle down and get used to the new kidney, as there are lots of things happening in your system.

Please note, the after care analysis in the book is for illustration and educational purposes only, and cannot replace the professional recommendations of doctors or consultants. Accurate analysis of the blood test results, and decisions to alter medication, is beyond the scope of this book.

**The tables are samples only; test results will vary for each individual. Also, high or low results on individual tests do not necessarily signify a reduction in kidney function, or possible rejection.

Conclusion

The problem of renal failure in developing countries, especially in African countries and communities is massive, and one that cannot be ignored, needing immediate and urgent attention. A lot of people die in African countries, due to ignorance associated with the sickness. In most cases, the sickness is not diagnosed on time, as some people still believe it is a taboo. This problem is a reality. When faced with renal failure, some people do not go to the right place for treatment. Some people start to sleep in churches; some go to dubious places to seek a solution, chasing shadows.

To treat a patient with kidney failure, costs include renal sessions, oral drugs and injections, such as the EPO injection, plus the cost of consultation. It is a massive cost, which a lot of individuals cannot afford; some will cut the number of their dialysis to once a week, or once every two weeks due to financial difficulty. This is not enough to get the blood properly cleansed. For a proper dialysis, you need to be dialysed three times a week. This inevitably leads to being vulnerable to a lot of physical problems and later, death.

Some that make it to the transplant stage do not stay the course, due to not being properly informed on how to live with a functioning graft; this is unfortunate.

There is no government subsidy in Third World countries, to help the less privileged pay for treatment. In the UK, the government takes care of the health of its citizens, as we have a system set up, and higher tax rate to help pay for this service. The government budgets a massive amount of money for health. That is why people like me are given the chance to live, despite my long years of sickness.

Additionally, too many people are not properly informed, and ignorant about the nature of their sickness, which parts 1 and 2 of my first book addresses. Some still do not believe in the existence of kidney failure. Some don't know how to cope with, or how to live with the sickness. They don't know who to talk to when they or a family member develops kidney failure. They don't know the causes, symptoms, or ways of detecting renal failure.

I stressed the importance of medical check-ups. These help detect unforeseen sickness. Some people in Third World countries do not believe in medical check-ups; some have never had a blood test in their entire life. They tend to put their trust in faith. They are ignorant of the situation. When you talk about medical check-ups, they believe that you are trying to bring sickness into them; they become emotional, and state that in the name of God they are not sick. They tend to confuse religious beliefs with the reality of life. Some have needlessly died out of this ignorance. Some have died within six months of their sickness, not being able to make it to the transplant stage.

Get a complete medical check-up done at least once in a year. Science has given us a lot of good things over the years. Please take the advantage of medical advances, for the good of your health...

I am an active supporter of introducing the UK system of the National Health Service to developing countries. It is the prime responsibility of each government to cater for the health of its people. A nation that is healthy and wealthy, is one where the government looks after the health concerns of its citizens.

My determination and will power, coupled with the power of my prayers, made me succeed in getting through this horrible sickness. Adopt a powerful attitude when you are going through, or recovering from any kind of sickness. You cannot give up. I was determined to succeed, and become well again.

I have emphasised the importance and power of prayer, but in conjunction with doing the right thing, i.e. getting proper, regular treatment. Science and religion work hand-in-hand. Do the right thing; go for your treatment, and then back yourself up with your prayers. Be careful how you use your religious beliefs. Have it both ways: practise your religion and back it up with God-given innovations of medical science.

I discussed the technical aspects of kidney transplantation, providing medical definitions, and details of various procedures, together with the positives and negatives of kidney transplantation. This is to broaden your understanding of the subject matter.

I also emphasised the importance of eating healthy to help with the recovery process, and avoiding excessive eating after the transplantation, as there is a tendency to put on excessive weight due to the steroids taken to prevent rejection. Too much weight can bring numerous unexpected health problems.

Taking medication on time and at the recommended dosage will help maintain a functioning kidney, and eliminate the problem of rejection.

I am of the opinion that we should educate Third World citizens by laying more emphasis on the importance of donating organs. We should encourage and teach the gift of life principle in our community, and also improve initiatives focused on best practises to increase the number of organs available for transplants. Everyone should be encouraged to join the donor register.

The role of after-care should not be undervalued, in helping to sustain a transplanted kidney. Blood tests should be often carried out so as to quickly detect the cases of rejection in new kidneys.

Governments should also support and encourage development and research into stem cell technology, and government funds should be channelled into this particular field of science. I am of the opinion that before long, we will witness the benefits this area of research will contribute to humanity.

******

Writing Living a Normal and Healthy Life After Renal (Kidney) Failure, parts 1 and 2, has been a pleasure.

Dear Reader, you are blessed for taking the time to read my book/s. May God continue to be with you, and support you. Amen.

I hope that you are now much more familiar with renal failure, with an increased awareness of all aspects of kidney transplantation.

GLOSSARY

Agitation – State of excessive psychomotor activity accompanied by increased tension and irritability.

Antibiotics – Substance produced by a semi-synthetic substance derived from a microorganism, and within a dilute solution, able to inhibit or kill other microorganisms.

Anticonvulsant drug – Medication used to control seizures

Biopsy – Hollow needle placed through the skin, withdrawing a sample from the tissue or organ to be examined.

Burn urine nitrogen. (BUN) – Measure, primarily of urea level in the blood.

Cardiovascular disease – Disease affecting the heart or blood vessels.

Convulsion – Abnormal violent involuntary contraction or series of contractions of the muscle.

Diagnose – To recognise (as a disease) by signs and symptoms.

Donor – Person used as a source a source of biological material (as blood or tissue).

ECG – Electrocardiogram- a simple, painless test for recording the heart's electrical activity.

ENT – Ear, nose and throat.

Enzymes – A complex protein produced by living cells, which breaks down food and other materials for assimilation in the body.

GP – General practitioner, doctor.

Hallucination – False sensory input (visual image or sound), can be caused by non-medicinal drugs, or a disorder of the nervous system.

Hypocalcaemia – Excess calcium in the blood.

Hypertension – Abnormally high arterial blood pressure.

Immune System – biological structures and processes within an organism that protects against disease by identifying and killing pathogens.

Listeria – Genus of small flagellated rod-shaped bacteria that do not form spores, aerobic, tendency to grow in chains, and include one which causes Listeria.

Neuropathic Pain – dysfunction within the nervous system.

Over-the-counter-medication – Drugs and medicine that may be sold without prescription.

Panel Redactive Antibody – Blood test done on patients waiting for a kidney transplant, which measures antibodies in the blood.

Pulmonary Infection – Occurs when normal lung or systematic defensive mechanism are impaired.

Renal Angiogram – an imaging test that uses x-rays to view blood vessels, to diagnose narrowed blood vessels to the kidney.

Renal Nephrologist – Renal doctor.

Surgical Procedure – Act of performing surgery.

Urinary Infection – bacterial infection that affects any part of the urinary tract — from which urine goes from the kidney via the bladder, out of the body.

REFERENCES

Please note that all web links are correct at the time of printing but may change over time.

Page

1. The science of prayer and healing, part 1 and 2, by Albert Einstein.

2, 3, 4, 5, 6, 7, 8, 9, 10, 11, 12, 13, 14, 15, 16, 17, 18, 19, 20, 21, 22, The Holy Bible, King James Version.

23, 24. www.lahey.org/medical/kidneytransplant/renaltransplants.asp

25. Lahey clinic. Select a medical service. Medical and surgical specialities. Types of renal transplants.

26. Department of Renal Medicine and Transplantation and the Pharmacy Department, Bart's, and London NHS Trust – prepared 28/07/08 – Mrs. Prima Nadesalingam.

27, 28, 29, 30, 31.
How the Spanish Donor System Works. By Branwen Jeffrey's, BBC News Health Correspondent, Madrid. Last updated 13 January, 2008.

32. Organ donor system overhaul. BBC home, last update 13 January, 2008.

33. http://news.bbc.co.uk/2/hi/health/7183559.stm
34. Journal of medical ethics. What's not wrong with conditional organ donation? http://jme.bmj.com/content/29/3/163.full
35. http://archive.student.bmj.com/issues/08/09/news/296.php

RESOURCES

UK

'NHS choices – Your Health, Your Choices: Kidney transplant.'

Kidney Research. UK Kidney Transplantation. www.kidneyresearchuk.org

Information on Living Donor Renal Transplants Addenbrooke Hospital NHS Trust, Transplant unit.

UK National Kidney Federation. Transplantation.

Primer on Transplantation, 2nd edition — Doug Norman, Laurence Turka. Wiley-Blackwell Publ.

Treatment Methods for Kidney Failure, Transplantation. National Institute of Diabetes, Digestive and Kidney Diseases (NIDDK) NIH.

Diet After a Renal Transplant – by Edren, Renal unit of Royal Infirmary of Edinburgh. www.edren.org/pages/edreninfo/diet-in-renal-disease/ diet-after-a-transplant.php

Addenbrooke Hospital NHS. Dietician's advice following renal transplant. www.cambridge-transplant.org.uk/ program/renal/diet.htm

BBC News – Health Transplant Goal One Step Closer. www.bbc.co.uk/2/hi/health/7205094.stm

Mouth Ulcers. British Health Foundation.

Cancer in the Mouth Can Affect You. NHS, June 2006. Cancer Research UK.

USA

Dialysis Versus Kidney Transplant. Medicine.net Health. Medical information produced by doctors. Visitor queries and doctors' response.

Kidney Transplant – Wikipedia. Free online encyclopaedia.

Post Operative Surgical Complications in Renal Transplant Proceedings, Volume 33, issue 5, pages 2683 – 2684.
H Karakayali.

We Bring Doctors' Knowledge to You. Definition of kidney transplant. www.medterms.com/script/main/art. asp?articlekey=6480

US National Library of Medicine. Medical Encyclopaedia — Kidney transplants. Reliable health information. www.medlineplus.gov

University of Maryland Transplant Centre, USA. Surgical webcast – Living Donor Kidney Transplant.

Kidney Transplantation – Symptoms, Treatment and Prevention. USA today. Health Encyclopaedia — diseases and conditions.

Diet after Transplantation – American Association of Kidney Patients. By Nikki, MS, RD, LD.
University of Southern California, Department of Surgery. Kidney transplant programme.
www.aakp.org/aakp-library/diet-after-transplantation

Healing Scriptures
www.alighthouse.com/phealingscripture.htm
christianfaith.blogspot.com/2009/03/prayers.for.sick.html
Prayers for Healing www.prayerguide.org.uk/prayer.htm
www.healingtherapies.info/prayer_and_healing.htm

Kidney Post Transplant Care, Life After Kidney
Transplantation. www.columbiakidneytransplant.org/life.
html

About medication after kidney transplant.
www.myfortic.com

Medicines that Prevent Rejection (Renal Life) By Thomas
G. Peter. MD, FACS www.aakp.org/aakp-library/
transplant-compatibility/index.cfm

Patient's Guide to Kidney Transplant Surgery
www.usckidneytransplantorg/patient guide/

WebMD, Living With an Organ Transplant. Diet and
weight gain. www.webmd.com/heart-disease/living-with-
an-organ-transplant/default.htm

Diet After Kidney Transplantation by Peggy Harum, RD,
CS, LD. Handout for patients with renal disease, written
by dietitians. www.nafwa.org/renal.php

Diet Therapy After Kidney Transplantation.
www.karger.com

Medicine Plus Dictionary. US Library of Medicine.
www.nlm.nih.gov/medlineplus/mplusdictionary.html

Health and medical information — doctor-produced, for
informed decisions on health issues.
www.medicinenet.com

ABOUT THE AUTHOR

Dr. Adeleke Eniola Oyenusi is a native of Irolu-Ijebu Remo, Ogun state, Nigeria. He attended the Methodist Primary School, Ekotedo, Ibadan, and later went to Holy Trinity Primary School, Ebute Ero, in Lagos. He left primary 5 in 1973 to continue his secondary school education from 1973 to 1977, gaining his basic certificate.

He briefly worked as a school teacher in 1977 at Ipara, after which he worked as a time keeper clerk at National Electric Power Authority in Sagamu, Nigeria. He completed his advanced level certificate in 1980 at the Remo Secondary School, in Sagamu. From 1980 to 1981 he worked as a wages clerk, at the Lagos State Transport Corporation.

In 1981, he moved to the former USSR, to study economics on a government scholarship. He then attended Kharkov University in the Ukraine, studying Russian for one year. After he proceeded to Minsk in 1982, to the Belarusian Institute of National Economy. As part of his Master's Degree in 1987, he had a job placement at the Federal Ministry of Planning, Ikoyi, Lagos. Having received his Master's Degree, he lived in Moscow, from October 1987 to 1992, completing his PhD in Economics, at the Russian Economic Academy.

Between 1992 and 1996 he worked as the Import Manager of Lake Pike Limited, Moscow, a company, which imported consumer goods.

He moved to London in 1996. On 26th December, 2000, he suffered a stroke that left him paralysed, but has since fully recovered. In 2002 he was diagnosed with end-stage renal failure. Initially he had a line treatment, then CAPD treatment and later haemodialysis. In 2008 he received a kidney transplant.

Dr. Adeleke Oyenusi is married to Gisele and has three children: Kimberlyne, Kelvin and Kenneth. He speaks English, Russian, French, Yoruba, Lingala and Ijebu.